Knee Pain in Sports Medicine

Knee Pain in Sports Medicine

Essentials of Diagnosis and Treatment

ANIS JELLAD
Department of Physical Medicine and Rehabilitation, Faculty of Medicine, University of Monastir and University Hospital of Monastir, Tunisia

AMINE KALAI
Department of Physical Medicine and Rehabilitation, Faculty of Medicine, University of Monastir and University Hospital of Monastir, Tunisia

AHMED ZRIG
Department of Radiology, Faculty of Medicine, University of Monastir and University Hospital of Monastir, Tunisia

ELSEVIER

Publisher: Sarah Barth
Acquisitions Editor: Humayra Khan
Editorial Project Manager: Sara Pianavilla
Production Project Manager: Selvaraj Raviraj
Cover Designer: Greg Harris

3251 Riverport Lane
St. Louis, Missouri 63043

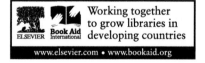

Working together
to grow libraries in
developing countries

www.elsevier.com • www.bookaid.org

Introduction

Nontraumatic knee injuries result from mild repetitive biomechanical stress associated with physical activity and exercise that exceeds the tissue tolerance and possibility of regeneration of the affected structure. They are also called microtraumatic injuries or overuse injuries. Repetitive forces applied to muscles, tendons, cartilage, or bones share the fact that they are of less energy than acute injury stresses [1].

The etiology of most knee overuse injuries is multifactorial, involving extrinsic factors (training errors) and intrinsic factors (anatomical and biomechanical variations).

The incidence of microtraumatic knee injuries is significant in athletes. A large number of knee injuries can be classified as overuse, accounting for 42% of all running injuries [1]. The prevalence of overuse injuries varies between sports activities [2].

The pathophysiology of knee overuse injuries will depend on the area and structures affected.

For example, traction forces increase stress in the patellofemoral joint by the transmission of abnormal loads through the articular cartilage and subchondral bone. Repetitive eccentric contraction of the knee extensor tendons while jumping is believed to be a cause of quadriceps and patellar tendinopathy (PT). Friction of the distal portion of the iliotibial band (ITB) over the lateral femoral epicondyle has been advanced in the pathogenesis of iliotibial band syndrome (ITBS) [3].

In the early stages of knee overuse disorders, the pain manifests while performing the predisposing activity and improves with rest, but in advanced stages, pain can be felt both during and after sports activities [4].

Development of chronic pain, impairment in sports performance or daily activities, and degenerative changes of the knee joint can occur when overuse injuries reach the chronic stage.

On rare occasions, some overuse injuries can lead to tendon rupture and may require surgical intervention.

Specific information about the sport and player position should be acquired. Recent changes in training techniques, training surfaces, shoes, stage of current training cycle, and next important competition should always be evaluated because these factors influence diagnosis, management, and prognosis.

Physical examination allows the clinician to identify predisposing biomechanical factors for microtraumatic knee injuries. These include femoral anteversion, knee valgus or varus, patellar malposition, static foot abnormalities, decreased strength of the vastus medialis muscle, and abnormal tracking of the patella [4].

Palpation for crepitation and pain in specific areas of the knee is necessary for the diagnosis. Muscles tightness and ITB should be evaluated.

Laboratory studies are not necessary for the diagnosis of knee overuse conditions. However, they should be included if other conditions, such as infection, malignancy, or inflammatory arthritis, are suspected.

Plain radiographs (weight-bearing anteriorposterior, lateral, and axial views) are not usually required as diagnostic tools, but they can help rule out other causes of knee pain.

In addition to its low cost, lack of radiation, and patient comfort when compared with other imaging modalities, ultrasonography (US) can be useful for the identification of focal changes in tendon architecture and subtle changes in tendon vascularity by using color Doppler [1,5].

Magnetic resonance imaging (MRI) can provide information about degenerative changes, subchondral bone edema, and cysts.

There are no specific treatment guidelines for most knee overuse injuries in sports. However, based on the nature of the disease process, review of the available medical literature, and expert clinical opinion, it is currently agreed that conservative therapy should be initially considered before surgical management in most conditions.

Nonsurgical treatment should include load reduction, correction of biomechanical abnormalities, strengthening and stretching exercises, pharmacological interventions, and physical modalities [6].

The role of specific rehabilitation programs of core and eccentric strengthening, modification of sport-specific techniques including foot strike mechanics in runners, and newer biological treatments, including platelet-rich plasma and the optimal surgery in patients who do not respond to conservative treatment, needs to be emphasized. The most frequently used physical agent is cryotherapy.

Antiinflammatory agents are the most common pharmacological agents used, including oral nonsteroid antiinflammatory drugs (NSAIDs) and local peritendinous injection of corticosteroids.

There are several emerging therapeutic interventions for knee overuse disorders. These include injection of platelet-rich plasma (PRP) [7,8] extracorporeal shockwave therapy [9,10], and stem cell therapy [11]. While some studies have shown promising results, there is a lack of randomized controlled trials supporting the use of this modality [12,13].

Surgical treatment is mainly based on clinical experience and expert opinion with weak to moderate quality studies.

Return to play is an important issue when dealing with athletic injuries. It is important to discuss this issue with the athlete and a multidisciplinary team, taking into consideration the athlete's competitive priorities and allowing for an informed decision to be made.

Despite their frequency and major consequences in athletes, there is a lack of pedagogic documents in the literature treating this group of knee conditions.

This work targeted physiatrists and residents in physical medicine and rehabilitation, orthopedics, and rheumatology specialities, as well as sports medicine practitioners.

This work will allow the user to:
- be able to establish the diagnosis for etiologies of knee pain of nontraumatic origin in athletes based on clinical examination and imaging modalities.
- formulate the differential diagnosis for these conditions.
- plan a multimodal multidisciplinary and adequate treatment strategy, involving the athletes, the team

doctors, and fitness trainers, that allows a prompt return to play and avoids recurrence of the condition.

REFERENCES

[1] Collado H, Fredericson M. Patellofemoral pain syndrome. Clin Sports Med 2010;29(3):379–98.

[2] Clarsen B, Bahr R, Heymans MW, Engedahl M, Midtsundstad G, Rosenlund L, et al. The prevalence and impact of overuse injuries in five N orwegian sports: application of a new surveillance method. Scand J Med Sci Sports 2015;25(3):323–30.

[3] Jelsing EJ, Finnoff JT, Cheville AL, Levy BA, Smith J. Sonographic evaluation of the iliotibial band at the lateral femoral epicondyle: does the iliotibial band move? J Ultrasound Med 2013;32(7):1199–206.

[4] Barry NN, McGuire JL. Overuse syndromes in adult athletes. Rheum Dis Clin North Am 1996;22(3):515–30.

[5] Hyman GS. Jumper's knee in volleyball athletes: advancements in diagnosis and treatment. Curr Sports Med Rep 2008;7(5):296–302.

[6] Fredericson M, Powers CM. Practical management of patellofemoral pain. Clin J Sport Med 2002;12(1):36–8.

[7] Fitzpatrick J, Bulsara M, Zheng MH. The effectiveness of platelet-rich plasma in the treatment of tendinopathy: a meta-analysis of randomized controlled clinical trials. Am J Sports Med 2017;45(1):226–33.

[8] Dragoo JL, Wasterlain AS, Braun HJ, Nead KT. Platelet-rich plasma as a treatment for patellar tendinopathy: a double-blind, randomized controlled trial. Am J Sports Med 2014;42(3):610–8.

[9] LLopis E, Padrón M. Anterior knee pain. Eur J Radiol 2007 Apr;62(1):27–43.

[10] Mani-Babu S, Morrissey D, Waugh C, Screen H, Barton C. The effectiveness of extracorporeal shock wave therapy in lower limb tendinopathy: a systematic review. Am J Sports Med 2015;43(3):752–61.

[11] Young M. Stem cell applications in tendon disorders: a clinical perspective. Stem Cells Int 2012;2012.

[12] Liddle AD, Rodríguez-Merchán EC. Platelet-rich plasma in the treatment of patellar tendinopathy: a systematic review. Am J Sports Med 2015;43(10):2583–90.

[13] Pas HI, Moen MH, Haisma HJ, Winters M. No evidence for the use of stem cell therapy for tendon disorders: a systematic review. Br J Sports Med 2017;51(13):996–1002.

Contents

CHAPTER 1

Patellofemoral Pain

1 BACKGROUND

Patellofemoral pain (PFP) can be defined as retropatellar or peripatellar pain resulting from physical and biochemical changes in the patellofemoral joint. It typically occurs with sport activity and often worsens when descending steps or hills or by prolonged sitting [1]. This term is used to describe painful symptoms located in the patellar region [1]. It is a very common complaint in the general population and particularly in young adult and adolescent athletes who participate in jumping and pivoting sports such as basketball, volleyball, and running [2]. It is reported that almost 25%–30% of all knee injuries seen in sports medicine and up to 40% of clinical visits in the general population for knee problems are related to PFP [3]. This syndrome is more frequent in female athletes and symptoms may cause sports cessation [4]. It has been reported to result in limitation of sport and physical activities in 74% of patients [5].

The physical examination has a key role in PFP diagnosis. It allows to investigate common risk factors such as patellar malalignment, muscular retractions, hip muscle weakness, poor core muscle endurance, and excessive foot pronation.

Imaging is not essential for the diagnosis of this condition and it is only needed in special cases.

Many possible interventions are recommended for PFP management. Due to the multifactorial nature of this syndrome, the clinical approach should be personalized.

In most cases, activity modification and rehabilitation are sufficient to limit the progression of symptoms. Therefore, they should be considered prior to surgical interventions.

2 SYNONYMS

- Anterior knee pain
- Anterior knee syndrome
- Patellofemoral pain syndrome
- Patellofemoral arthralgia
- Chondromalacia patellae
- Lateral patellar compression syndrome
- Patellalgia

A recent consensus statement from the Fourth International Patellofemoral Pain Research Retreat recommended PFP as the preferred term [6].

3 CLINICAL STUDY

3.1 Symptoms

History in athletes presenting with PFP may reveal recent modifications in sport activities including changes in the frequency, duration, and intensity of training [7]. The training program should also be evaluated for errors including a rapid increase in exercise intensity, inadequate recovery time, and extreme uphill or downhill running [8]. A history of similar symptoms indicate that the condition is chronic and is presenting as an acute exacerbation [7]. The use of inappropriate or excessively worn footwear, recent heavy resistance training and running on altered surface or hills should also be considered.

A history of knee traumatic injuries, including patellar subluxation or dislocation, or surgeries should be noted, as they may directly damage the articular cartilage or change the forces across the patellofemoral joint, resulting in PFP [8].

Patients with PFP typically describe vague pain behind, underneath, or around the patella. This pain usually appears with activities such as squatting, running, and use of stairs [8]. If asked to point to the site of pain, patients may place their hands over the anterior aspect of the knee or draw a circle with their fingers around the patella. This sign is known as the circle sign and is suggestive of PFP.

The onset of symptoms is usually gradual. The pain may be unilateral or bilateral and is usually described as dull, but may be sharp [8]. Sometimes, patients report stiffness or pain on prolonged sitting with the knees flexed. This is known as the theater sign [7].

Patients may occasionally report knee instability concomitant to the pain occurrence due to quadriceps muscle inhibition, or locking while going from knee extension to flexion, and a feeling of a popping or grinding can be present [8].

Knee Pain in Sports Medicine. https://doi.org/10.1016/B978-0-323-88069-5.00009-3

3.2 Physical Examination

A physical examination is the key to PFP diagnosis, but there is no single conclusive clinical test [9]. A variety of tests have been advanced to diagnose this condition.

3.2.1 Vastus medialis coordination test

The patient lies supine, the examiner places his fist under the subject's knee and asks the patient to extend the knee slowly. The patient is instructed to achieve full extension. The test is considered positive when a lack of coordinated full extension is apparent, that is, when the patient either has difficulty to smoothly achieve extension or uses the extensors or flexors of the hip to accomplish extension. A positive test may be an indicator of dysfunction of the vastus medialis obliquus muscle [10] (Fig. 1.1).

3.2.2 Patellar apprehension test or smillie test

The patellar apprehension test is performed with the patient in supine position. The examiner uses one hand to push the patient's patella as lateral as possible. Starting with the knee flexed at 30 degrees, the examiner grasps the leg at the ankle with the other hand and performs a slow flexion of the knee and hip. The lateral patellar slide is maintained throughout the test. A positive test consists of orally expressed apprehension or an apprehensive quadriceps recruitment [11] (Fig. 1.2).

3.2.3 Eccentric step test

This test requires the use of a step that is 15 cm high or more accurately with a height equal to 50% of the length of the patient's tibia. The patient is asked to stand on the step, put the hands on the chest, and step down

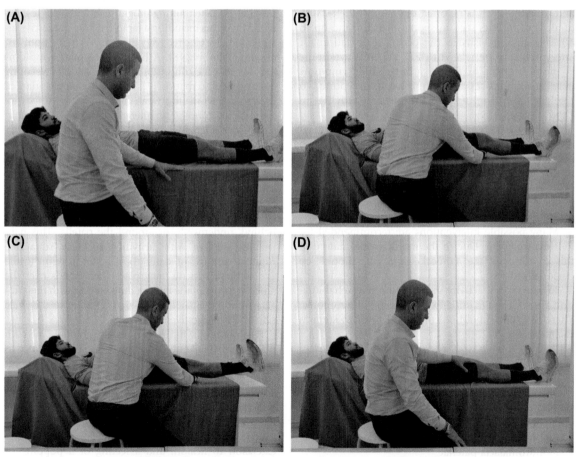

FIG. 1.1 Pictures illustrating the vastus medialis coordination test: (A) Starting position: The patient lies supine with his knee extended. (B) The examiner places his fist under the patients' knee resulting in a slight flexion. (C) The examiner instructs the patient to perform knee extension. (D) Final position: the patient relaxes his knee extensors and returns to the resting position.

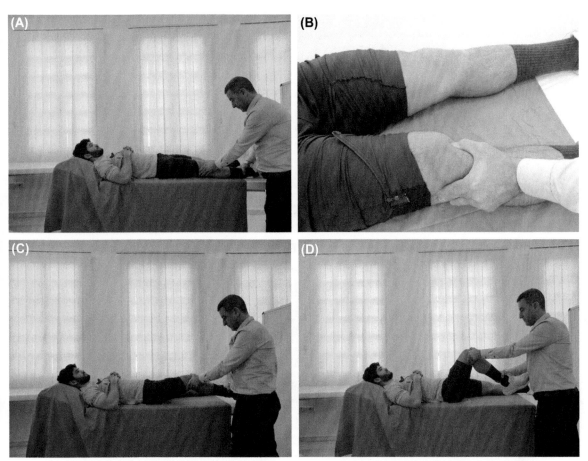

FIG. 1.2 Pictures illustrating the patellar apprehension test or smillie test. (A) Starting position: the patient lies supine with his knee extended and the examiner places his thumb on the medial edge of the patella. (B) The examiner uses one hand to push the patient's patella as lateral as possible. (C) The examiner places the knee at 30 degrees flexion while maintaining the lateral pressure on the patella. (D) The examiner performs combined knee and hip flexion while maintaining lateral pressure on the patella.

as slowly and smoothly as possible. The patients should keep the hands on the chest throughout the test performance. The eccentric step test is considered positive when the patient reports knee pain during the test performance [12].

3.2.4 Waldron's test (Phases I and II)
To do Phase I of Waldron's test, the patient lies supine and the examiner presses the patella against the femur while performing a passive knee flexion with the other hand. For Phase II, the standing patient performs a slow, full squat, again with the examiner performing a gentle compression of the patella against the femur. In both phases, crepitus and pain are considered signs of PFP disorders [13].

3.2.5 Clarke's test or patellofemoral grinding test or Zohlen's test
The grinding test is performed with the patient lying supine. The examiner presses the patella distally (with the hand on the superior border of the patella) and then requests the patient to contract the quadriceps muscle. The test will be considered positive if the patient's pain is reproduced [13] (Fig. 1.3).

3.2.6 Standard step-down test
Standard step-down test is very similar to eccentric step test, except that the patient should stand with arms on the hips and be instructed to squat down 5–10 times consecutively in a slow and controlled manner until the heel touches the floor, maintaining

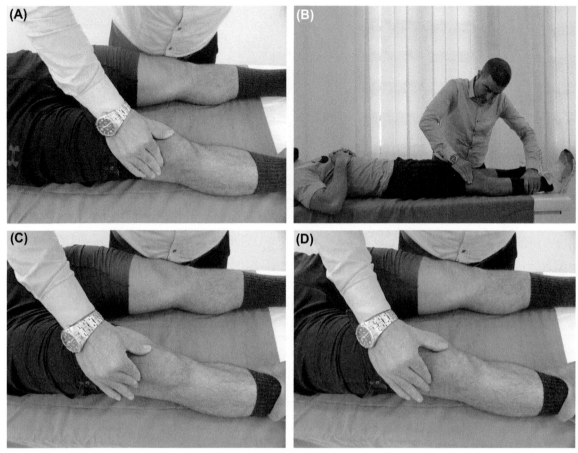

FIG. 1.3 Pictures illustrating Clarke's test or patellofemoral grinding test or Zohlen's test. (A) Starting position: The patient lies supine while the examiner locates the proximal end of the patella. (B) The examiner applies downward pressure on the patella. (C) The examiner asks the patient to contract his quadriceps muscle. (D) Finishing position: The patient relaxes his quadriceps muscle while the examiner removes the pressure on the patella.

his balance at a rate of approximately one squat per 2 s. Scoring of the deviations in the trunk, pelvis, hip, and knee reveals the onset timing of the anterior gluteus medius, hip abduction torque, and decreased lateral trunk strength [13].

Excellent interrater and intrarater reliability has been reported for this test [12].

In addition to these tests, the clinical evaluation should include hip muscle strength evaluation looking for a misbalance between hip internal rotators/external rotators and hip abductors/adductors and podoscopic examination of the feet looking for over pronation since these abnormalities have been described as risk factors for PFP [6] (Fig. 1.4).

4 DIFFERENTIAL DIAGNOSIS

Differential diagnosis of PFP includes other causes of anterior knee pain.

4.1 Plica Syndrome

The main symptom of plica syndrome is knee pain localized to the anterior aspect of the knee that is worsened when using stairs, squatting, or bending and a catching or a locking sensation can be felt when extending the knee.

4.2 PT

Pain in the anterior aspect of the knee is the first symptom of patellar tendinopathy (PT). This pain is

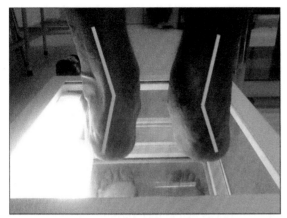

FIG. 1.4 Picture illustrating bilateral foot over pronation on podoscopic examination in a patient with PFP.

- Patients older than 50 years (to assess for patellofemoral osteoarthritis).
- Patients who are skeletally immature (to rule out other causes such as physeal injury or bone tumors).
- Suspected cases of bipartite patella, loose bodies and occult fractures.
- Patients who do not demonstrate improvement after several weeks of conservative treatment.

In these cases, weight-bearing anterior-posterior, lateral, and axial views should be performed [8].

Standard anterior-posterior radiograph is useful for differential diagnosis, allowing to identify degenerative joint disease and bone tumors [8].

The lateral view is most valuable for patellar height assessment (Fig. 1.5).

Axial views allow the evaluation of degenerative changes in the patellofemoral joint, patellar morphology, dysplasia of the trochlear groove, and ectopic calcifications in the retinaculum [7] (Fig. 1.6).

5.2 Computed Tomography

Computed tomography (CT) scan is not needed for the majority of patients with PFP. The axial views are helpful to evaluate the trochlear groove. This imaging modality is also highly sensitive to femoral alignment and femorotibial rotation and is usually indicated in cases where surgical treatment is planned.

5.3 Magnetic Resonance Imaging

Magnetic resonance imaging (MRI) is the best tool to evaluate patellar malalignment, trochlear dysplasia, patellar tilt, and articular chondral injuries [14].

worsened by sports activities that require knee extension. On physical examination, there is tenderness on the proximal insertion of the patellar tendon.

4.3 Sinding—Larsen—Johansson Syndrome

Pain localized to the inferior patellar pole in a young athlete with swelling is suggestive of SLJS.

4.4 Patellar Dislocations

A history of acute knee trauma and joint effusion is frequently found.

4.5 Osgood—Schlatter Disease

Tenderness and swelling around the tibial tuberosity in adolescents is suggestive of Osgood—Schlatter disease (OSD).

4.6 Patellar Instability or Subluxation

Sensations of the patellar movement or popping out may suggest patellar instability or subluxation, mainly during rotational activities.

4.7 Systemic Rheumatologic Joint Disease

Prolonged morning stiffness, simultaneous involvement of several joints or tendons, and joint swelling may be a presentation of systemic rheumatologic joint disease.

5 IMAGING

5.1 Standard X-rays

The diagnosis of PFPS is mainly clinical. However plain radiography may be indicated in the following cases:
- A history of recent trauma, dislocation or surgery, joint effusion.

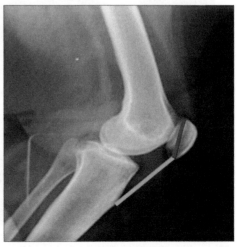

FIG. 1.5 Knee lateral view standard X-ray showing a patella alta in a patient with PFP.

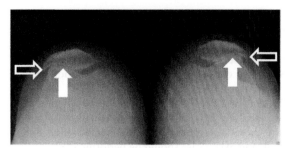

FIG. 1.6 Axial radiograph of the knees showing a dysplasia of the trochlear grooves with narrowing of the patellofemoral joint (*stars*) and lateral osteophytes of the patella (*arrows*) in both knees in a patient with PFP.

Cartilage loss, subchondral sclerosis, edema, and cystic changes at the patellar and trochlear surfaces are the main MRI findings in case of PFP [15] (Figs. 1.7 and 1.8).

MRI can be useful in detecting loose bodies, patellar stress fractures, and bone marrow edema, which is suggestive of patellar subluxation or dislocation [8].

6 TREATMENT

6.1 Conservative Treatment
There is general agreement that nonsurgical interventions are the primary choice for PFP treatment.

6.1.1 Activity modification
In professional athletes, the impact of rest will be more evident than in recreational sportsmen. In an acute

injury, relative rest will allow the tissue to heal and the symptoms will be reduced. Athletes should be advised to avoid prolonged sitting positions, squatting, and lunges and reduce the intensity of exercises that put a load on the knee in flexion. Running shoes should be adapted and training on unsteady surfaces should be avoided.

6.1.2 Medical treatment
Drugs commonly used for PFP include simple analgesics such as paracetamol and nonsteroidal antiinflammatory drugs (NSAIDs). The latter may not be adapted to the treatment of this condition due to the absence of a histologic inflammatory manifestation in many PFP cases as well as their possible adverse effects on normal healing response of muscles and tendons. Short courses of NSAIDs may be helpful when other modalities such as exercise and analgesics have failed to control pain.

6.1.3 Rehabilitation
There is consistent evidence that exercise therapy for PFP results in important reduction of pain and improvement in functional capacities.

Combining hip and knee exercises is more successful to reduce pain and improve function and this combination should be preferred to knee exercises alone [16].

Both strengthening and stretching exercises are recommended in rehabilitation therapy. Assessment of individual risk factors may determine the proper combination of different exercises [17]. A special importance should be given to neuromuscular exercises

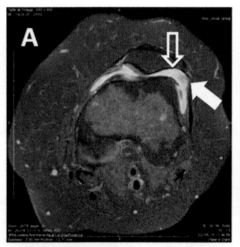
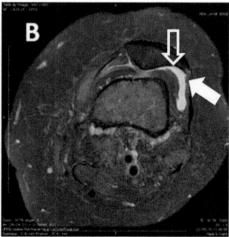

FIG. 1.7 MRI axial sections of the right knee without Gadolinium injection in Proton Density (A) and FAT SAT (B) showing extensive carilaginous lesions of the lateral facet of the patella with exposure of the subchondral bone (*red arrows*). The patella are eccentred with trochleo-patellar dysplasia. An intraarticular effusion (*star*) and lateral retinaculum lesion (*green arrow*) are also present.

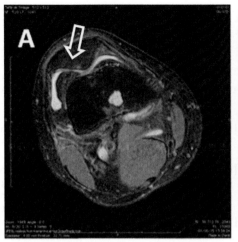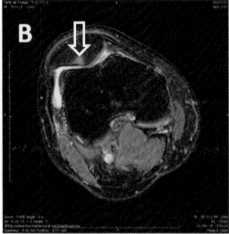

FIG. 1.8 MRI axial sections of the right knee of a 38-year-old patient with PFP, without Gadolinium injection, in DP (A) and FAT SAT (B) showing extensive carilaginous lesions of the medial facet of the patella with exposed subchondral bone and edema of the subchondral bone (*arrows*), an eccentred patella and minimal intraarticular effusion.

since their efficacy in treating patients with PFP has been proved.

Positive results were achieved with strengthening exercises, particularly knee extension, squats, stationary cycling, static quadriceps contractions, active straight-leg raise, leg press, and step-up and step-down exercises.

Stretching of the hamstring, quadriceps, iliopsoas, gastrocnemius, and iliotibial band (ITB) muscles has been found to be useful for PFP treatment. Studies found that lower extremity stretching alone or combined with strengthening exercises may improve PFP symptoms in up to 60% of patients [18].

Cryotherapy is a physical agent that is recommended as a part of the conservative treatment for PFP for pain management [19].

The Gundersen Health System Sports Medicine Rehabilitation Program for PFP is an evidence-based program that allows patients to return to sports-related activities as quickly and safely as possible. Individual variations will be made based on patient tolerance and response to treatment (Annex 1).

6.1.4 Orthoses

Static foot abnormalities should be corrected with foot orthoses since they can influence knee biomechanics.

There is moderate evidence that knee braces have additional benefit over exercise therapy on pain and function. Thus patellar braces should only be used as an adjunct to other interventions.

6.2 Procedures

Corticosteroid injections are recommended if local inflammatory signs (especially an effusion) are present and provide short to medium term pain relief.

Hyaluronic acid injections can be used in patients with radiologic signs of patellofemoral osteoarthritis.

Acupuncture and dry needling have been suggested for the treatment of PFP, but few studies found a statistically significant pain reduction following acupuncture [19]. Sclerotherapy and prolotherapy injections are also suggested with positive results [19]. There is some evidence that Botulinum toxin type A injection to the distal region of vastus lateralis muscle may increase vastus medialis activation [20]. Patellofemoral, knee, and lumbar mobilization or manipulation have been proposed as alternatives, but are not recommended according to the current evidence [18].

A multimodal approach is highly recommended to reduce pain in athletes with PFP in the short and medium terms [18].

6.3 Surgical Treatment

Surgery is the last resort for PFP and appears to be inadequate. Open, arthroscopic, and percutaneous techniques have been described as surgical options.

These techniques include lateral retinacular release to decrease lateral traction force, proximal and distal realignment procedures, and elevation of the tibial tubercle.

Surgery is usually reserved for refractory cases that do not respond to conservative treatment. In carefully selected patients, surgery may be successful, although failure rates of 20%–30% have been reported [19].

In some selected cases such as serious malalignment, patella alta or lateral patellar compression syndrome, good outcomes have been reported [21].

TAKE HOME MESSAGES

PFP is a frequent cause for presentation at physical medicine and rehabilitation, general practice, orthopedic and sports medicine clinics in particular.

Several intrinsic and extrinsic risk factors have been reported and should be investigated and corrected.

A thorough clinical examination based on specific clinical tests is the cornerstone to diagnose PFP.

Standard X-rays are useful for eliminating differential diagnosis. CT scan and MRI are helpful for evaluating patellar and trochlear morphology.

A multimodal conservative intervention including exercise therapy, activity modification, and minimally invasive procedures is commonly sufficient to manage PFP patients.

REFERENCES

[1] Witvrouw E, Werner S, Mikkelsen C, Van Tiggelen D, Berghe LV, Cerulli G. Clinical classification of patellofemoral pain syndrome: guidelines for non-operative treatment. Knee Surg Sports Traumatol Arthrosc 2005; 13(2):122–30.

[2] Loudon JK, Gajewski B, Goist-Foley HL, Loudon KL. The effectiveness of exercise in treating patellofemoral-pain syndrome. J Sport Rehabil 2004;13(4):323–42.

[3] Kannus P, Aho H, Järvinen M, Nttymäki S. Computerized recording of visits to an outpatient sports clinic. Am J Sports Med 1987;15(1):79–85.

[4] Nimon G, Murray D, Sandow M, Goodfellow J. Natural history of anterior knee pain: a 14-to 20-year follow-up of nonoperative management. J Pediatr Orthop 1998; 18(1):118–22.

[5] Fairbank JC, Pynsent PB, van Poortvliet JA, Phillips H. Mechanical factors in the incidence of knee pain in adolescents and young adults. J Bone Joint Surg Br 1984; 66(5):685–93.

[6] Doberstein ST, Romeyn RL, Reineke DM. The diagnostic value of the Clarke sign in assessing chondromalacia patella. J Athl Train 2008;43(2):190–6.

[7] Dixit S, Difiori JP, Burton M, Mines B. Management of patellofemoral pain syndrome. Am Fam Physician 2007;75(2):194–202.

[8] Collado H, Fredericson M. Patellofemoral pain syndrome. Clin Sports Med July 2010;29(3):379–98.

[9] Nunes GS, Stapait EL, Kirsten MH, de Noronha M, Santos GM. Clinical test for diagnosis of patellofemoral pain syndrome: systematic review with meta-analysis. Phys Ther Sport 2013;14(1):54–9.

[10] Nijs J, Van Geel C, Van de Velde B. Diagnostic value of five clinical tests in patellofemoral pain syndrome. Man Ther 2006;11(1):69–77.

[11] Malanga GA, Andrus S, Nadler SF, McLean J. Physical examination of the knee: a review of the original test description and scientific validity of common orthopedic tests. Arch Phys Med Rehabil 2003;84(4):592–603.

[12] Selfe J, Harper L, Pedersen I, Breen-Turner J, Waring J. Four outcome measures for patellofemoral joint problems: part 1. Development and validity. Physiotherapy 2001;87(10):507–15.

[13] Myrtos CD. Conservative management of sports injuries. J Can Chiropr Assoc June 2012;56(2):157.

[14] Duran S, Cavusoglu M, Kocadal O, Sakman B. Association between trochlear morphology and chondromalacia patella: an MRI study. Clin Imag 2017;41:7–10.

[15] Elias DA, White LM. Imaging of patellofemoral disorders. Clin Radiol 2004;59(7):543–57.

[16] Crossley KM, van Middelkoop M, Callaghan MJ, Collins NJ, Rathleff MS, Barton CJ. 2016 Patellofemoral pain consensus statement from the 4th International Patellofemoral Pain Research Retreat, Manchester. Part 2: recommended physical interventions (exercise, taping, bracing, foot orthoses and combined interventions). Br J Sports Med 2016;50(14):844–52.

[17] Halabchi F, Mazaheri R, Mansournia MA, Hamedi Z. Additional effects of an individualized risk factor–based approach on pain and the function of patients with patellofemoral pain syndrome: a randomized controlled trial. Clin J Sport Med 2015;25(6):478–86.

[18] Crossley K, Bennell K, Green S, McConnell J. A systematic review of physical interventions for patellofemoral pain syndrome. Clin J Sport Med April 2001;11(2):103–10.

[19] Hiemstra LA, Kerslake S, Irving C. Anterior knee pain in the athlete. Clin Sports Med July 2014;33(3):437–59.

[20] Singer BJ, Silbert BI, Silbert PL, Singer KP. The role of botulinum toxin type a in the clinical management of refractory anterior knee pain. Toxins August 25, 2015;7(9): 3388–404.

[21] AL-Sayyad MJ, Cameron JC. Functional outcome after tibial tubercle transfer for the painful patella alta. Clin Orthop March 2002;396:152–62.

CHAPTER 2

Patellar Tendinopathy

1 BACKGROUND

Patellar tendinopathy (PT) is a common syndrome encountered in sports medicine. The symptoms are located in the distal extremity of the patella or in the proximal patellar tendon [1] (Fig. 2.1).

They can be intense and lead to stoppage of sports activity.

This condition is related to sports that involve frequent jumping such as volleyball and basketball, which explains why this condition is also called jumper's knee [2].

Repetitive jumping results in a considerable pressure on the knee extensor mechanism. The main pathophysiologic phenomenon in PT is tendinosis, which is a degenerative rather than an inflammatory disorder. Therefore, the use of the term tendinitis is not appropriate to describe this injury.

Prevalence of PT in professional volleyball players has been reported to be at 45% and 32% in professional basketball players [2]. In other sports, such as soccer, in which jumping is not the main activity, PT has been reported in up to 2.4% of players [3].

PT has been reported to have extrinsic and intrinsic risk factors. They include anthropometric factors, such as a high body mass index, a large abdominal circumference, limb-length difference, and flat foot [4]. Biomechanical factors such as weak quadriceps muscles and inextensibility or tightness of the quadriceps and hamstring muscles are also associated with PT. Gender and some factors associated with the sport itself, including the training surface, were not found to be correlated with the development of PT [4].

Patients typically present with an activity-related anterior knee pain that is precisely localized to the distal pole of the patella and the proximal end of the patellar tendon. The onset of the pain is usually insidious.

The diagnosis is mainly clinical, but imaging is needed when the symptoms are not typical.

The conservative management of PT is commonly sufficient to relieve symptoms. Surgical treatment is indicated for refractory cases.

2 SYNONYMS

Patellar tendinitis
　Patellar tendinosis
　Patellar chondropathy
　Partial rupture of patellar ligament

3 CLINICAL STUDY

3.1 Symptoms

Patients with PT usually report a well-localized anterior knee pain that is related to the intensity of activity [1].

Pain is usually insidious and aggravates gradually. It may be precipitated by an increase in the frequency or intensity of repetitive extension movements of the knee.

Initially, pain may present as a dull ache at the beginning of sports activities or after their accomplishment. This initial symptom may be ignored as it disappears during the activity [5]. With continued use, however, pain can progress to be present during activity and interfere with performance significantly.

In some cases, there is a constant painful sensation at rest and at night that alters sleep [6].

Other common complaints are pain with prolonged sitting and when using the stairs [7].

3.2 Physical Examination

On clinical examination, the most frequent finding is patellar tendon tenderness [7]. This tenderness is typically located at the inferior pole of the patella that is influenced by knee position [8]. With the knee flexed to 90°, the tendon is placed under tension, and tenderness significantly decreases and may disappear altogether so the patellar tendon should be palpated in relaxed full-knee extension or with slight knee flexion (Fig. 2.2).

Mild isolated pain should not be given much significance as it may be a normal finding in active athletes [9].

Stretching and resisted contraction of the quadriceps may reproduce the patient's usual pain (Fig. 2.3).

Knee Pain in Sports Medicine. https://doi.org/10.1016/B978-0-323-88069-5.00004-4

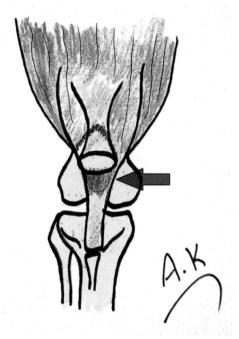

FIG. 2.1 Drawing showing the location of inflammation at the patellar tendon's proximal insertion point (*arrow*).

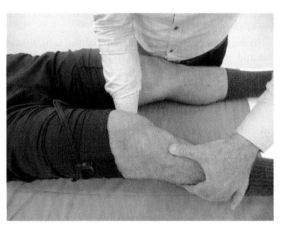

FIG. 2.2 Picture illustrating patellar tendon palpation in slight knee flexion position.

Patients with chronic symptoms may exhibit weakness of the quadriceps, with the vastus medialis obliquus portion being the most commonly affected.

Functional strength testing of the quadriceps may be performed by asking the patient to perform one-legged step-downs [10]. The strength of the calf can be assessed by performing single-legged heel raises. A jumping athlete should be able to perform a minimum of 40 raises [10]. During both activities, the onset of fatigue and the quality of movement should be monitored and both activities should be performed bilaterally.

To reproduce PT symptoms, a useful functional test is the decline (30 degrees) squat test. This test places greater load on the patellar tendon than does a squat on level ground [10]. The objective measurement during this test can be obtained by determining the number of decline squats before the onset of pain and asking the athlete to indicate the level of pain on a visual analog or verbal reporting scale. An alternative method of objectively assessing an athlete with PT is to use the Victorian Institute of Sport Assessment scale [11]. This scale provides a numerical index of the severity of PT by assessing both pain and function. A maximum score of 100 indicates full, pain-free function (Annex 2).

4 DIFFERENTIAL DIAGNOSIS

4.1 Retinacular Pain

Patients with patellofemoral malalignment frequently complain of dull aching or pain in the anterior knee that is worsened by patellar retinaculum tensioning.

4.2 Fat Pad Lesion

The patient presents with pain on either side of the patellar tendon, where the fatty tissue sits. The pain may be worse with jumping, prolonged standing, or any other position with knee hyperextension. Besides, the area around the patellar tendon may be slightly swollen. Fat pad impingement is not associated with clicking, locking, or instability.

4.3 Lipoma Arborescens

This condition is characterized by an insidious onset of painless swelling of the affected joint, usually persisting for many years, followed by progressive pain accompanied by intermittent episodes of joint effusion.

4.4 Infrapatellar Bursitis

Symptoms of bursitis commonly include swelling and anterior knee pain that is worsened with flexion and usually occurring at night or after activity.

4.5 Partial Anterior Cruciate Ligament (ACL) Tear

A certain degree of laxity is found on ligamentous laxity tests of the knee.

4.6 Entrapment of the Saphenous Nerve

The patient usually complains of pain in the anteromedial aspect of the knee. The physical examination

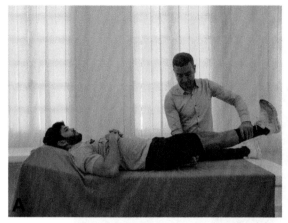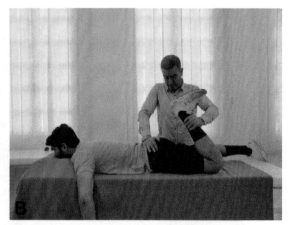

FIG. 2.3 Pictures illustrating quadriceps muscle resisted contraction (A) and stretching (B).

reveals a positive Tinel's sign on the medial aspect of the knee and pressure over this area reproduces the patient's pain.

5 IMAGING

5.1 Standard X-rays

The use of radiographs during initial evaluation is limited since radiographic changes are rarely present during the first six months of PT evolution [4].

When radiography is performed, the examination generally includes anteroposterior, lateral, and sunrise patellar views [3].

Possible findings include radiolucency at the tip of the patella and an elongation of the involved pole. On occasions, calcification of the involved tendon and irregularity or avulsion of the patellar pole may be seen in the late stages [1].

5.2 Ultrasound

Ultrasound (US) provides an available, quick, and inexpensive method of imaging for the patellar tendon.

In suspected PT cases, US can be used to confirm the existence and location of intratendinous lesions. These lesions are reflected by decreased echogenicity, typically in the deep posterior portion of the tendon adjacent to the lower pole of the patella [12].

Other common findings on US include tendon thickening, irregularity of the tendinous envelope, intratendinous calcification, and erosion of the patellar tip [12].

It has been shown that there is no correlation between the severity of tendinopathy symptoms on clinical grading systems and tendon appearance on US [13].

5.3 Magnetic Resonance Imaging

On magnetic resonance imaging (MRI), PT is characterized by a focal increase in signal within the tendon as well as an alteration in its size [14].

Increased thickening of the patellar tendon on MRI is present in all patients resistant to conservative therapy. An anteroposterior diameter of 7 mm has been suggested as a limit between symptomatic and asymptomatic tendons (Fig. 2.4).

The main disadvantages of MRI are its relatively high cost, limited availability in some regions, and the long time required for scanning.

6 TREATMENT

6.1 Conservative Management

Most authors agree that initial management should be conservative rather than surgical. This agreement is based on the fact that time of recovery with appropriate conservative management is equivalent to the one following surgery and that the outcome of conservative management is equal to the outcome following surgery [2].

Physicians should keep in mind that recovery can be prolonged taking 4−6 months in chronic cases [2]. In athletes with a short duration of symptoms, recovery to full sporting capacity may take 2−3 months [2]. Professional athletes need special attention as they may be able to warm up the injury, resulting in full sporting capacity, further mechanical overload, and further tendon degeneration. RICE protocol (Rest, Icing, Contention, and Elevation) should be followed during the initial management of this tendinopathy.

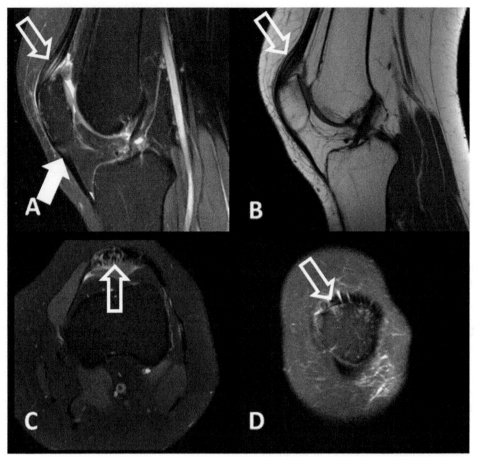

FIG. 2.4 MRI sections of the right knee without Gadolinium injection, in sagittal DP FAT SAT (A) and T1 (B), axial (C) and coronal DP FAT SAT (D) demonstrating significant fusiform thickening of the quadriceps tendon (*red arrows*) and patellar tendon (*green arrows*) in relation to quadricipital and patellar tendinopathy. Note the absence of intraarticular effusion.

6.1.1 Activity modification

Initial conservative management should involve some form of load reduction to limit progression of the pathology.

Given the negative effects of complete immobilization, load reduction should be achieved by relative rest rather than complete stopping of activity.

Relative rest means that the athlete may be able to continue playing or training with modification of pain-provoking activities and reduction in total training hours.

In addition to changing training activities and durations, lower limb biomechanical correction can reduce patellar tendon loading by improving its energy-absorbing capacity. A biomechanical correction includes training on how to land from a jump so that greater energy is absorbed by distal and proximal joints and not the knee [15].

6.1.2 Medical treatment

Antiinflammatory medications are the most common pharmacological treatments used in PT especially oral nonsteroidal antiinflammatory drugs (NSAIDs) and corticosteroids. The use of both has been debated, considering that tendinopathy has a noninflammatory mechanism.

6.1.3 Rehabilitation

Research has shown that soft-tissue mobilization promotes healing. Thus, massage therapy is used in PT to promote repair and to decrease adhesions between the tendon fibers [7].

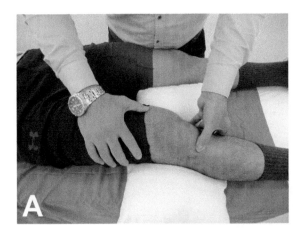
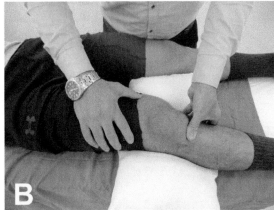
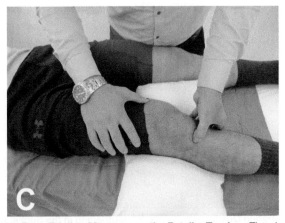

FIG. 2.5 **Pictures Illustrating Deep Friction Massage on the Patellar Tendon.** The physiotherapist locates the patellar tendon and applies direct pressure (A), while maintaining the pressure on the patellar tendon, the physiotherapist performs transversal friction movements (B and C).

The most effective form of massage appears to be digital pressure followed by deep transverse friction throughout the entire tendon [7] (Fig. 2.5).

Massage should also be performed on both the calf and quadriceps muscles to maintain their flexibility [7].

In PT, hamstring and quadriceps tightness and weakness need to be managed [14]. As the rehabilitation program advances and pain decreases, eccentric strengthening exercises should be emphasized (Figs. 2.6 and 2.7).

These types of strengthening exercises are optimal for rehabilitation of tendinopathies because they place the maximal tension load on the muscle and tendon unit [16]. It should be noticed that these types of exercises may initially provoke pain, given the increased load placed on the muscle-tendon unit.

The final phase of rehabilitation should also include sports-specific movements and training. Knee braces and straps have been used to alleviate pain and to change the force dynamics through the patellar tendon with good results [4].

Initial exercises should focus on strength and endurance gains before progressing to speed gains.

Pain should guide the strengthening activity intensity, and during all exercises, the quality of movement should be given importance.

A range of electrophysical modalities have been employed to treat PT. These include US, laser, and electrical stimulation.

US and laser can stimulate collagen production and increase mechanical strength during repair of acute tendon injuries [17].

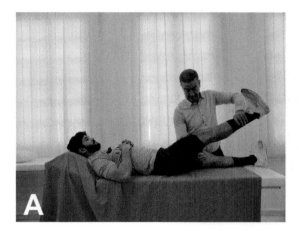
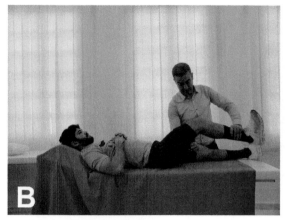
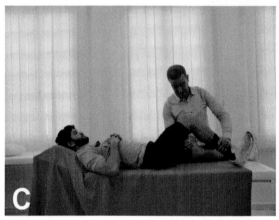

FIG. 2.6 **Pictures Illustrating Quadriceps Muscle Strengthening in the Supine Position.** The patient lies supine with his knee extended (A), performs an eccentric quadriceps contraction (B) and finish in the rest position.

Icing may have a role in the management of PT, particularly after strengthening exercises. It reduces blood flow and may help to reduce the pathological neovascularization associated with tendinopathy [12].

6.1.4 Orthoses
Forces on the knee may also be influenced by foot mechanics, and thus shoe orthoses may be indicated in some athletes with static foot abnormalities.

6.2 Procedures
Peritendinous corticosteroid injection could have beneficial effects by reducing connective tissue and peritendinous adhesions (Fig. 2.8).

This injection may be performed with US guidance to ensure accurate placement of the needle. Decreased pain with injection of the fat pad has been reported [3].

6.3 Surgical Treatment
Surgery for PT is only indicated after failure of a well-established 6-month conservative treatment program.

Surgery may include excision of degenerated areas, arthroscopic debridement, repair of macroscopic defects, multiple longitudinal tenotomies, drilling of the inferior pole of the patella, resection of the tibial attachment of the patellar tendon with realignment, percutaneous needling, or percutaneous longitudinal tenotomy [7].

The exact surgical technique chosen is based on the surgeon's opinion and experience.

A review found that the outcome following surgery was either excellent or good in 46%−100% of cases, with a maximum success rate of 75%−85% [18]. Thus, 15%−25% of patients will experience persistent or recurrent tendon pain after surgery.

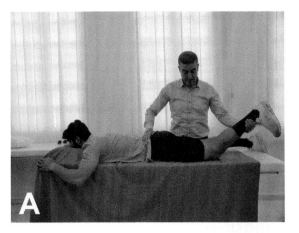
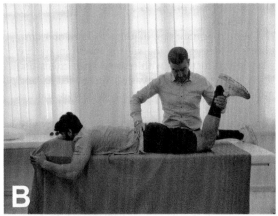
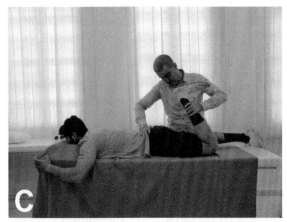

FIG. 2.7 **Pictures Illustrating Quadriceps Muscle Strengthening in the Prone Position.** The patient lies prone and is instructed to resist the knee flexion performed by the physiotherapist (A), the resistance is carried out through the complete flexion range of motion (B and C).

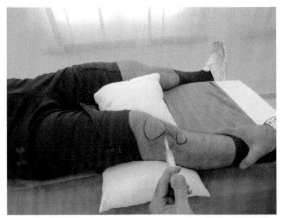

FIG. 2.8 Picture showing the placement of the needle for corticosteroid injection in case of PT.

Recovery after surgery can take up to six to twelve months and some athletes will not be able to return to their previous level of sport even with good surgical results. Consequently, surgery should only be performed after failure of an implemented thorough conservative management program.

7 TAKE HOME MESSAGES

PT is a chronic overuse injury of the patellar tendon resulting from excessive biomechanical stress on the knee extensor mechanism.

Athletes involved in sports requiring repetitive jumping, running, and kicking are highly exposed to developing this syndrome (Jumper's knee).

Patients typically report a dull anterior knee pain that is insidious in onset. It is commonly well localized and initially appears only after an intense sport activity or competition.

The most important sign of jumper's knee on examination is tenderness at the site of insertion on the patellar tip that increases with resisted knee extension.

US is inexpensive, noninvasive, reproducible, and examination sensitive allowing early diagnosis and dynamic imaging of the tendon.

Conservative treatment is a key choice in the management of jumper's knee. However, surgery is indicated in the chronic stage.

REFERENCES

[1] Khan KM, Cook JL, Kannus P, Maffulli N, Bonar SF. Time to abandon the "tendinitis" myth. BMJ March 16, 2002; 324(7338):626−7.

[2] Lian OB, Engebretsen L, Bahr R. Prevalence of jumper's knee among elite athletes from different sports: a cross-sectional study. Am J Sports Med April 2005;33(4):561−7.

[3] Hägglund M, Zwerver J, Ekstrand J. Epidemiology of patellar tendinopathy in elite male soccer players. Am J Sports Med September 2011;39(9):1906−11.

[4] van der Worp H, van Ark M, Roerink S, Pepping GJ, van den Akker-Scheek I, Zwerver J. Risk factors for patellar tendinopathy: a systematic review of the literature. Br J Sports Med April 2011;45(5):446−52.

[5] Sandmeier R, Renström PA. Diagnosis and treatment of chronic tendon disorders in sports. Scand J Med Sci Sports April 1997;7(2):96−106.

[6] Khan KM, Bonar F, Desmond PM, Cook JL, Young DA, Visentini PJ, et al. Patellar tendinosis (jumper's knee): findings at histopathologic examination, US, and MR imaging. Victorian Institute of Sport Tendon Study Group. Radiology September 1996;200(3):821−7.

[7] Khan KM, Maffulli N, Coleman BD, Cook JL, Taunton JE. Patellar tendinopathy: some aspects of basic science and clinical management. Br J Sports Med December 1998; 32(4):346−55.

[8] Warden SJ, Brukner P. Patellar tendinopathy. Clin Sports Med October 2003;22(4):743−59.

[9] Cook JL, Khan KM, Kiss ZS, Purdam CR, Griffiths L. Reproducibility and clinical utility of tendon palpation to detect patellar tendinopathy in young basketball players. Victorian Institute of Sport tendon study group. Br J Sports Med February 2001;35(1):65−9.

[10] Cook JL, Khan KM, Maffulli N, Purdam C. Overuse tendinosis, not tendinitis part 2: applying the new approach to patellar tendinopathy. Phys Sportsmed June 2000;28(6): 31−46.

[11] Visentini PJ, Khan KM, Cook JL, Kiss ZS, Harcourt PR, Wark JD. The VISA score: an index of severity of symptoms in patients with jumper's knee (patellar tendinosis). Victorian Institute of Sport Tendon Study Group. J Sci Med Sport January 1998;1(1):22−8.

[12] Fritschy D, de Gautard R. Jumper's knee and ultrasonography. Am J Sports Med December 1988; 16(6):637−40.

[13] Lian Ø, Holen KJ, Engebretsen L, Bahr R. Relationship between symptoms of jumper's knee and the ultrasound characteristics of the patellar tendon among high level male volleyball players. Scand J Med Sci Sports October 1, 1996;6(5):291−6.

[14] Yu JS, Popp JE, Kaeding CC, Lucas J. Correlation of MR imaging and pathologic findings in athletes undergoing surgery for chronic patellar tendinitis. Am J Roentgenol July 1, 1995;165(1):115−8.

[15] Richards DP, Ajemian SV, Wiley JP, Zernicke RF. Knee joint dynamics Predict patellar tendinitis in elite volleyball players. Am J Sports Med September 1, 1996;24(5): 676−83.

[16] Blazina ME, Kerlan RK, Jobe FW, Carter VS, Carlson GJ. Jumper's knee. Orthop Clin N Am July 1973;4(3): 665−78.

[17] Enwemeka CS. The effects of therapeutic ultrasound on tendon healing. A biomechanical study. Am J Phys Med Rehabil December 1989;68(6):283−7.

[18] Coleman BD, Khan KM, Maffulli N, Cook JL, Wark JD. Studies of surgical outcome after patellar tendinopathy: clinical significance of methodological deficiencies and guidelines for future studies. Scand J Med Sci Sports February 1, 2000;10(1):2−11.

CHAPTER 3

Quadriceps Tendon Injuries

1 BACKGROUND

Microtraumatic quadriceps tendon injuries usually include conditions ranging from tendinosis to partial thickness tears to complete tendon rupture and less commonly recalcitrant tendinitis.

These lesions are relatively uncommon in painful knee conditions [1]. In fact, in sports medicine practice, quadriceps tendinopathy is less common than the patellar one [2]. Quadriceps tendinopathy and especially rupture should be kept in mind when investigating acute symptoms associated with the extensor mechanism of the knee [3].

The quadriceps is a strong part of the extensor system of the knee, but it can be affected by degenerative changes, under the influence of local and systemic factors leading to tendinopathy and in some cases to spontaneous, partial, or complete rupture. For this reason, prevention and treatment of predisposing factors and early recognition can be helpful in identifying patients susceptible to rupture [1].

Practicing regular sport activity in advanced ages and weight lifting sports are considered risk factors for quadriceps tendinopathy. Quadriceps tendon is biomechanically exposed to heavy loads stress and microtrauma resulting from deep squat exercises and sudden acceleration forces [4].

Patients usually report an insidious onset of knee pain especially located at the superior pole of the patella. On examination of the knee, tenderness in the tendon insertion, painful resisted contraction and stretching allow to establish the diagnosis of tendinopathy.

All grades of quadriceps tendinopathy are usually treated conservatively. Conservative treatments include extracorporeal shock waves as well as autologous growth factors injection which are particularly effective [3].

2 SYNONYM

Quadriceps tendinosis.

3 CLINICAL STUDY

3.1 Symptoms

Quadriceps tendinopathy may interfere with daily activities. Pain is usually felt when climbing the stairs, kneeling, and rising from a chair. Athletes may be unable to participate in running and jumping activities [1].

Patients usually report an insidious onset of knee pain and may notice painful clicking. A burning sensation at the bone-tendon junction may be experienced [4].

The pain is aggravated by activities resulting in load stress of the extensor mechanism, including bending, stair climbing, running, and jumping.

Reports of severe weakness are alarm features suggesting the possibility of a quadriceps tendon partial or complete rupture.

The quadriceps tendon rupture is more common in older subjects (>50 years) with associated systemic factors, such as obesity, gout, and local degenerative changes such as knee osteoarthritis [5]. Patients with tendon ruptures are unable to walk without assistance and usually hold their leg as straight as possible.

The investigator should look for a history of renal insufficiency, primary or secondary hyperparathyroidism, diabetes, rheumatoid arthritis, gout, use of quinolones, corticosteroid injections, and anabolic steroids and obesity which impair and weaken the osteotendinous junction [6−8]. Furthermore, a genetical predisposition is incriminated in case of bilateral rupture of the quadriceps tendon [9].

3.2 Physical Examination

On examination of the knee, tenderness is localized along the superior pole of the patella and the quadriceps tendon.

Pain in the quadriceps tendon area may be reproduced by extreme knee flexion and by resisted knee extension (Fig. 3.1).

The clinician should also look for a palpable defect, suggesting partial or complete rupture of the quadriceps tendon.

Knee Pain in Sports Medicine. https://doi.org/10.1016/B978-0-323-88069-5.00014-7

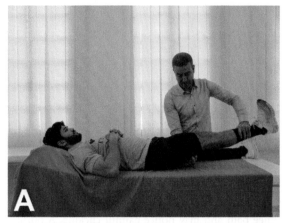 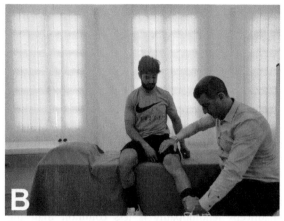

FIG. 3.1 Pictures showing a resisted knee extension test. The patient attempts to extend the knee, while the examiner exerts an opposing force. Patient in supine position (A) and sitting on the table border (B).

Neurologic examination findings are usually normal. Painful weakness is related to complete or partial tendon rupture. Stability of the knee is typically not affected.

Usually, a localized tenderness and thickening along the course of the tendon are clinically present.

Jolles et al. proposed a minimally invasive test that can clinically determine the integrity of the quadriceps tendon in its five distal centimeters, which was inspired by the O'Brien test for complete rupture of the Achilles tendon [9]. With the patient lying in the supine position, in aseptic condition, a 25-gauge needle is inserted in a right angle through the skin of the thigh, at a midline point, 5 cm proximal to the superior pole of the patella. The needle is inserted gently through the skin until greater resistance is felt, so that the needle's tip is just within the substance of the quadriceps tendon but without transfixing it.

A passive knee flexion and extension movement is then performed, and the movement of the needle is observed. Two distinct types of response may occur. If the needle pivots about its penetration point in the skin, the tendon is intact throughout its distal 5 cm. If the needle does not pivot (positive test), this indicates loss of continuity of the quadriceps tendon between its insertion and the position of the needle [9].

Despite these clinical signs, misdiagnosis is frequent, ranging from 39% to 67% [2].

4 DIFFERENTIAL DIAGNOSIS

4.1 Patellar Tendinopathy

Pain and tenderness are located next to the distal pole of the patella.

4.2 Patellar Fracture

A history of a direct trauma on the kneecap is usually found. Radiographic findings confirm the diagnosis.

4.3 Patellofemoral Syndrome and Chondromalacia Patellae

Pain is felt as retropatellar or peripatellar. It typically occurs with activity and often worsens when descending the stairs or hills or by prolonged sitting. Dull, aching pain, and/or a feeling of grinding when the knee is flexed are typically present in case of chondromalacia patellae.

4.4 Prepatellar Bursitis

Swelling in the peripatellar region alongside with pain in the anterior aspect of the knee are suggestive of prepatellar bursitis.

5 IMAGING

5.1 Standard X-rays

Standard radiographs may have some diagnostic value for quadriceps tendinopathy and tendon tears. In the chronic stage of tendinopathy, they may show calcifications suggesting a recalcitrant tendinopathy. The abolition of the quadriceps shadow, the presence of a mass in the suprapatellar soft tissues secondary to tendon retraction, and the avulsion of a bony segment from the proximal pole of the patella are all typical radiographic features of tendon rupture. The low-riding patella or patella baja is another feature suggestive of quadriceps tendon rupture.

5.2 Ultrasound

The ultrasound (US) examination is a more effective method for diagnosing tendinopathy and rupture of the quadriceps tendon compared to traditional radiography [8].

Thickening of the different layers and loosening of the fibrillar structure are pathognomonic signs of degenerative tendon disease [10].

The US images of quadriceps tendinopathy can be extremely heterogeneous, from some degenerative alterations limited to a single layer of the tendon, to larger ones involving the whole tendon. In the first case, tendinopathy can be recognized as a hypoechogenic oval image while in the second one, a wider hypoechogenicity of the different collagen layers will be described.

Calcifications may be present in some cases and a pathologic hypervascularization phenomenon is seen in the acute stage.

The previous US findings are sometimes present in asymptomatic individuals and are considered as risk factor for the occurrence of painful symptoms in the future [11].

5.3 Magnetic Resonance Imaging

Magnetic resonance imaging (MRI) is an important instrumental method for quadriceps tendon evaluation. It is recommended before any surgical treatment [12].

In case of partial rupture, at least one of the layers is still intact. The superficial layer is the most common site of injury, followed by the intermediate one [13] (Fig. 3.2).

When a total rupture occurs, there is an interruption of all the tendon layers, with a possible hematoma in the area of the lesion. In this case, MRI demonstrates a retracted proximal stump and a wavy look of the patellar tendon [2].

In dynamic MRI, by the traction of the patella, it is possible to observe an increase in the interval between the two tendon stumps.

6 TREATMENT

6.1 Conservative Treatment

The RICE protocol should be followed for the initial management of this tendinopathy especially in the acute phase.

6.1.1 Activity modification

A conservative management of this condition should include relative rest with modification of pain-provoking activities and a reduction in total training hours to limit progression of the pathology. Complete stoppage of sports activity should be avoided given its negative effects.

Lower limb biomechanical correction can reduce quadriceps tendon loading by improving its energy-absorbing capacity.

6.1.2 Medical treatment

Analgesics such as paracetamol may be useful to reduce painful symptoms especially in the acute stage. Antiinflammatory medications are among the most common pharmacological treatments used in quadriceps tendinopathy, especially oral nonsteroidal antiinflammatory drugs (NSAIDs) and corticosteroids. The use of both has been debated considering that tendinopathy has a noninflammatory mechanism.

6.1.3 Rehabilitation

Quadriceps tendinopathy is responsive to the same physiotherapy treatments of patellar tendinopathy (PT) [14].

Deep friction massage, US, and extracorporeal shock wave therapy (especially in case of calcifications) represent valid physical modalities for treating quadriceps tendinopathy [15].

Eccentric exercises play a key role in the conservative treatment of this tendinopathy. Dimitrios et al. [16] demonstrated that the combination of eccentric training and quadriceps stretching exercises would be superior to eccentric training alone, in order to reduce pain and improve function (Fig. 3.2).

Isometric exercises should be implemented early in the rehabilitation program since they have been associated with an immediate effect in controlling pain in tendinopathies, with sustained effect for at least 45 min, allowing an increase in quadriceps strength [17] (Fig. 3.3).

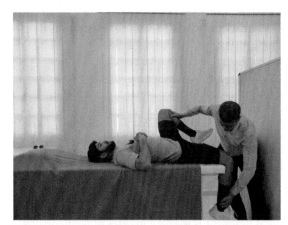

FIG. 3.2 Picture illustrating a stretching technique of the quadriceps muscle in the supine position.

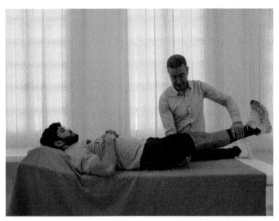

FIG. 3.3 Picture illustrating a resisted isometric contraction of the quadriceps muscle.

The rehabilitation program will also include exercises aimed to recover the range of motion (ROM). Rehabilitation treatment is also very important after surgery as ROM exercises are needed for patients who undergo delayed repair due to loss of full knee flexion and decreased quadriceps strength [18].

6.1.4 Orthoses
Forces on the knee may also be influenced by foot mechanics, and thus foot orthoses may be indicated in some athletes with static foot abnormalities.

6.2 Procedures
6.2.1 PRP injection
Nowadays, the use of platelet-rich plasma (PRP) has become very popular in tendon and muscle repair. This has been tried in quadriceps tendinopathy and partial ruptures with good results [19]. The mechanism of action seems to be related to reduction of inflammation and increased collagen synthesis [20].

6.2.2 Corticosteroid injection
The use of injectable corticosteroids has been tried in the treatment of quadriceps tendinopathy in order to reduce inflammation and pain and to positively interfere with the altered tendon tissue, but it is not supported by strong clinical evidence given the associated risk of tendon rupture [21].

7 SURGICAL TREATMENT
Surgical treatment is required in cases of tendinopathy that resist to conservative management and in full thickness tendon tears.

The earlier the injury is diagnosed, the better the prognosis of surgical treatment will be. Technical evolution of surgical materials has enabled an improvement in terms of functional results [22].

Surgical techniques for quadriceps tendon repair are different. Generally, for midsubstance ruptures, end-to-end sutures are used, while patellar drilling or anchors are largely used in ruptures closer to the osteotendinous junction.

Augmentation techniques are applied in the presence of poor quality of tendon tissue or in case of delayed surgery and when a quadriceps retraction is present.

The viscoelastic properties of tendons and muscles determine the degree of retraction during the rupture process. Thus, surgeons should work on preserving the original tendon length since inadequate muscle function will persist if the retracted quadriceps becomes too short to function properly.

After surgery, according to the biological processes of tendon healing and some clinical evidence, six weeks seems to be the most appropriate period of immobilization. After this period, it is essential to plan a proper and customized rehabilitative program for functional and strength recovery of the knee in order to prevent and avoid joint stiffness and functional impairment [14].

8 TAKE HOME MESSAGES
Quadriceps tendon is biomechanically exposed to heavy loads stress and microtrauma resulting from deep squat exercises and sudden acceleration forces which are substratum for tendinopathy.

Pain and tenderness in the superior pole of the patella are the most frequent symptoms.

Early recognition and prevention of predisposing factors are helpful to protect athletes from ruptures.

US and MRI contribute to the diagnosis of quadriceps tendinopathy and are sensitive for detecting tendon tears.

Quadriceps tendinopathy treatment is mainly conservative, and it is based on rehabilitation, physical therapies such as extracorporeal shockwave therapy, and autologous growth factors injection.

Surgical techniques for quadriceps tendon repair are different depending on the rupture location. Generally, end-to-end sutures are used for midsubstance ruptures, while patellar drill holes or anchors are largely used in ruptures close to the osteotendinous junction.

Postsurgical rehabilitation is crucial in order to preserve tendon and muscle viscoelastic proprieties and recover adequate knee extensor mechanism function.

REFERENCES

[1] La S, Fessell DP, Femino JE, Jacobson JA, Jamadar D, Hayes C. Sonography of partial-thickness quadriceps tendon tears with surgical correlation. J Ultrasound Med Off J Am Inst Ultrasound Med December 2003;22(12): 1323−9. quiz 1330−1.

[2] Tuong B, White J, Louis L, Cairns R, Andrews G, Forster BB. Get a kick out of this: the spectrum of knee extensor mechanism injuries. Br J Sports Med 2011; 45(2):140−6.

[3] Abram SG, Sharma AD, Arvind C. Unusual association of diseases/symptoms: Atraumatic quadriceps tendon tear associated with calcific tendonitis. BMJ Case Rep 2012;2012.

[4] Brukner P. Brukner & Khan's clinical sports medicine. McGraw-Hill North Ryde; 2012.

[5] Kumar S, Rachakatla N, Kerin C, Kumar R. Simultaneous traumatic rupture of the patellar tendon and the contralateral quadriceps tendon in a healthy individual. BMJ Case Rep 2010;2010.

[6] Maffulli N, Del Buono A, Spiezia F, Longo UG, Denaro V. Light microscopic histology of quadriceps tendon ruptures. Int Orthop 2012;36(11):2367−71.

[7] Ilan DI, Tejwani N, Keschner M, Leibman M. Quadriceps tendon rupture. JAAOS-J Am Acad Orthop Surg. 2003; 11(3):192−200.

[8] Fhoghlu CN, Ellanti P, Moriarity A, McCarthy T. MRI features of a quadriceps tendon rupture. BMJ Case Rep 2015; 2015.

[9] Jolles BM, Garofalo R, Gillain L, Schizas C. A new clinical test in diagnosing quadriceps tendon rupture. Ann R Coll Surg Engl 2007;89(3):259−61.

[10] PICCIN Nuova Libraria S.P.A. Ultrasonografia del sistema muscoloscheletrico. Available from: http://www.piccin.it/it/ortopedia/1739-ultrasonografia-del-sistema-muscoloscheletrico-9788829920631.html.

[11] Visnes H, Tegnander A, Bahr R. Ultrasound characteristics of the patellar and quadriceps tendons among young elite athletes. Scand J Med Sci Sports 2015;25(2):205−15.

[12] Swamy G, Nanjayan S, Yallappa S, Bishnoi A, Pickering S. Is ultrasound diagnosis reliable in acute extensor tendon injuries of the knee?. 2012.

[13] Yu JS, Popp JE, Kaeding CC, Lucas J. Correlation of MR imaging and pathologic findings in athletes undergoing surgery for chronic patellar tendinitis. Am J Roentgenol July 1, 1995;165(1):115−8.

[14] Kountouris A, Cook J. Rehabilitation of Achilles and patellar tendinopathies. Best Pract Res Clin Rheumatol 2007;21(2):295−316.

[15] Wang CJ. Extracorporeal shockwave therapy in musculoskeletal disorders. J Orthop Surg 2012;7(1):11.

[16] Dimitrios S, Pantelis M, Kalliopi S. Comparing the effects of eccentric training with eccentric training and static stretching exercises in the treatment of patellar tendinopathy. A controlled clinical trial. Clin Rehabil 2012;26(5): 423−30.

[17] Rio E, Kidgell D, Purdam C, Gaida J, Moseley GL, Pearce AJ, et al. Isometric exercise induces analgesia and reduces inhibition in patellar tendinopathy. Br J Sports Med 2015;49(19):1277−83. bjsports-2014.

[18] Matava Null. Patellar tendon ruptures. J Am Acad Orthop Surg November 1996;4(6):287−96.

[19] Molloy T, Wang Y, Murrell GA. The roles of growth factors in tendon and ligament healing. Sports Med 2003;33(5): 381−94.

[20] Júnior N, Cavalcanti A, Júnior M de JM. The effects of laser treatment in tendinopathy: a systematic review. Acta Ortopédica Bras 2015;23(1):47−9.

[21] Loppini M, Maffulli N. Conservative management of tendinopathy: an evidence-based approach. Muscles Ligaments Tendons J 2011;1(4):134.

[22] Maniscalco P, Bertone C, Rivera F, Bocchi L. A new method of repair for quadriceps tendon ruptures. A case report. Panminerva Med 2000;42(3):223−5.

CHAPTER 4

Iliotibial Band Syndrome

1 BACKGROUND

Iliotibial band syndrome (ITBS) is a common cause of lateral knee pain in athletes. This syndrome was first described in 1975 as a condition affecting US Marine recruits, who undergo rigorous endurance training [1]. The number of cases diagnosed with ITBS has increased with the growing popularity of recreational distance running and cycling. Epidemiologic studies have identified ITBS as the most common cause of lateral knee pain in runners. Its incidence has been reported to range from 1.6% to 12% [2,3]. Among cyclists, ITBS is held responsible for 15%–24% of all overuse injuries [3]. ITBS symptoms have also been reported in competitive rowers, skiers, and athletes participating in soccer, basketball, triathlons, and field hockey [4–6].

Patients with ITBS may also present with a lateral snapping hip. This sign is related to the ITB rapidly passing anteriorly over the greater femoral trochanter. Athletes sometimes report an audible painful snap on landing from a jump [7].

The etiology of ITBS is still not clearly defined. Suggested theories include:
- Compression of the fat and connective tissue deep to the ITB.
- Chronic inflammation of the iliotibial bursa.
- Friction of the ITB against the lateral femoral epicondyle during repetitive flexion and extension activities (Fig. 4.1).

The diagnosis is typically made based on patient history and physical examination with specific tests to assess the ITB for tightness and to reproduce the patient's symptoms.

Several risk factors have been identified. Training errors, including rapid changes in training routine, hill running, and increased distances are commonly cited [8,9]. The surface of activity can also contribute to the development of ITBS in runners, as running on inclined surfaces can put excessive stress on the lateral compartment of the knee. Downhill running tends to be worse because of the decrease in knee flexion at the time of foot strike increasing the forces exerted on the knee [10,11].

The anatomic factors that contribute to increased tension of the ITB and lateral knee strain include excessive genu varum, excessive internal tibial rotation, foot pronation, hip abductor weakness, and paralytic disorders which result in muscle imbalance [8].

2 SYNONYM

Iliotibial band friction syndrome.
  Runner's knee.
  Iliotibial tract friction syndrome.
  Snapping knee.

3 CLINICAL STUDY

3.1 Symptoms

On initial consultation, patients with ITBS usually report pain situated on the lateral aspect of the knee. Typically, they localize the pain precisely in the region of the distal ITB, between the lateral femoral condyle and its insertion on the Gerdy tubercle (Fig. 4.2).

In the early stages of the disease, the symptoms usually occur at the completion of a repetitive flexion-extension exercise. As the condition worsens, pain is often experienced earlier in the athletic activity and may be present at rest.

Questions about the patient's history include the distance run or cycled per week, condition of the athlete's running shoes, the presence of swelling, and mechanical symptoms and aggravating/relieving factors. The patients usually report an increase in symptom frequency and intensity when running outside, when running down hills, and when increasing stride length [11].

3.2 Physical Examination

A complete knee examination is imperative in order to identify ITBS and to rule out other pathologies representing the differential diagnosis of lateral knee pain.

Static lower extremity alignment must be evaluated. The examiner should look for varus of the knee which increases the ITB tension.

Knee Pain in Sports Medicine. https://doi.org/10.1016/B978-0-323-88069-5.00012-3

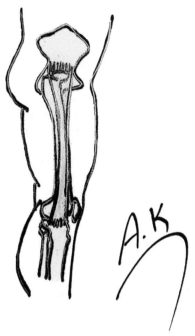

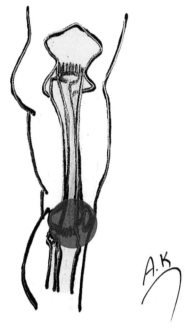

FIG. 4.1 Anatomy of the iliotibial band, which can cause snapping as it slips anteriorly and posteriorly over the prominent greater trochanter and lateral femoral condyle.

FIG. 4.2 Drawing illustrating the pain location and radiation in patients with ITBS (red circle).

The knee should be examined for evidence of an effusion or soft-tissue swelling.

ITBS patients often present with tenderness at the level of the lateral femoral condyle, approximately 3 cm proximal to the knee joint.

While palpating the lateral femoral epicondyle throughout knee flexion and extension, Renne [1] described a sound similar to rubbing fingers on a wet balloon and Noble [8] described the sound like wet leather.

A complete ligament examination should be performed and knee range of motion (ROM) should be assessed and typically no abnormalities should be found.

Four tests are commonly used in the assessment of ITB function and ITBS diagnosis.

3.2.1 Renne's test

While standing on the involved side, the patient is instructed to place one hand on the examiner's shoulder for balance and slowly squat (one legged) to 60—90 degrees flexion and then rise back up. The test is

considered positive if it reproduces the patient's pain (Fig. 4.3).

3.2.2 The Noble test

This test is performed with the patient lying supine, beginning with the affected knee flexed at 90 degrees and the leg is extended with direct pressure over the lateral femoral epicondyle. The test is positive when pain is reproducible near 30 degrees of knee flexion [8] (Fig. 4.4).

3.2.3 The Ober test

The Ober test can be used to assess ITB tightness. With the patient lying on his side with the unaffected leg down and bent at 90 degrees, the examiner stabilizes the pelvis, then abducts and extends the affected leg. Then, the examiner tries to adduct the leg. The Ober test is positive when the examiner cannot adduct the affected leg from this position [12] (Fig. 4.5).

3.2.4 The Thomas test

This test is used to evaluate the tightness of the iliopsoas muscle, rectus femoris muscle, and ITB. The patient is instructed to lie supine at the edge of the examination

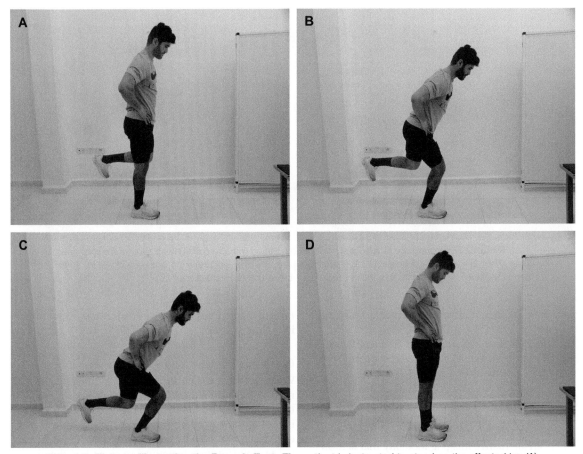

FIG. 4.3 **Pictures Illustrating the Renne's Test.** The patient is instructed to stand on the affected leg (A), then perform slow controlled knee flexion (B), then slow controlled knee flexion (C), and finish with rest position both feet on the ground (D).

table with both knees held to the chest. While the examiner stabilizes the pelvis, the patient holds the unaffected leg to the chest, and the affected leg is extended and lowered. The test is considered positive when the patient cannot completely extend and lower the affected leg horizontally [13] (Fig. 4.6).

4 DIFFERENTIAL DIAGNOSIS

Differential Diagnosis of ITBS includes:

1. Lateral meniscal tear
   In this case, meniscal tests are positive.
2. Lateral compartment degenerative joint disease
   Joint line tenderness and knee radiographs allow the diagnosis.

3. Biceps femoris (BF) tendinopathy
   Tendinous tests are positive.
4. Stress fracture
   Knee radiographs usually show the fracture line.
5. Patellofemoral pain
   Knee pain is mainly localized on the anterior aspect of the knee.

5 IMAGING

5.1 Standard X-rays

Anteroposterior, lateral, and sunrise views should be performed. They can be used to rule out other possible causes of lateral knee pain, such as lateral joint space

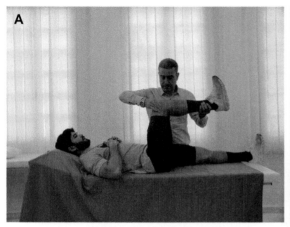
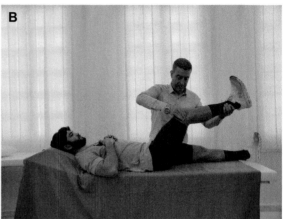

FIG. 4.4 **Pictures Illustrating the Noble Test.** Starting position with the patient lying supine, the examiner flexes the affected knee at 90 degrees and applies direct pressure over the lateral femoral epicondyle (A), then he extends the knee while maintaining the pressure over the lateral femoral condyle (B).

narrowing from osteoarthritis, patellar maltracking, and stress fractures.

The iliotibial tract can sometimes be identified on anteroposterior radiograph of the lower extremity as a vertical linear soft-tissue opacity [14].

5.2 Ultrasound

Ultrasound (US) is an excellent imaging modality for superficial soft tissues, including ITB [15]. In general, US offers an alternative imaging modality that is more convenient and cost-effective than magnetic resonance imaging (MRI). It also allows for ITB dynamic assessment [16].

On sonographic examination, ITB is a relatively hyperechoic linear structure that has a fibrillar pattern. Proximally, it can be easily visualized in the axial plane as a band over the greater trochanter [17].

Around the knee, ITB can be seen in the coronal plane, with the distal insertion at Gerdy's tubercle, and in the axial plane over the lateral femoral epicondyle [15]. The use of dynamic US examination at the greater trochanter and lateral femoral epicondyle can be used to demonstrate sudden movement of ITB over these bony structures as the cause of snapping hip or snapping knee syndrome [18].

Its use is recommended in the follow-up of patients with the diagnosis of ITBS because of the low cost and availability of this modality compared with MRI [19].

5.3 CT Scan

On computed tomography (CT) imaging, the iliotibial tract will be a hyperdense structure relative to adjacent muscular structures. This examination has a low value in the diagnosis of ITBS.

5.4 Magnetic Resonance Imaging

When definitive diagnosis is needed or other diagnoses need to be excluded, MRI can be used as a diagnostic tool. The presence of a high-intensity signal representing a fluid-filled collection over the lateral epicondyle deep to the ITB as well as a marked thickening and partial tearing (intrinsic hyperintense signal) of the distal ITB has been reported [20].

MRI can also be useful in ruling out other potential causes of lateral knee pain, including articular cartilage injuries, meniscal tears, and cysts.

6 TREATMENT

6.1 Conservative Management

6.1.1 Activity modification

Rest from the culprit activity is indicated. When pain resolves, a gradual return to activity may help to avoid symptom recurrence.

In cycling, equipment modification such as changing cleat position or lowering the bicycle seat and raising the handlebars may decrease pain and allow for an early return to activity [21].

6.1.2 Medical treatment

Oral nonsteroidal antiinflammatory drugs (NSAIDs) and corticosteroid can be administered to reduce the acute inflammatory response.

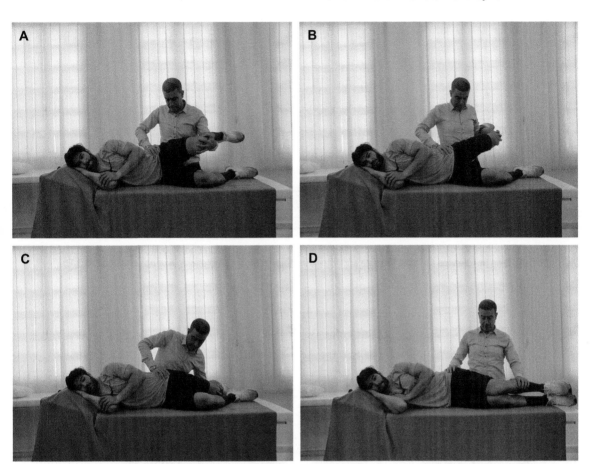

FIG. 4.5 **Pictures Illustration the Ober Test.** While the patient lies on the unaffected side with his knees and hips flexed, the examiner stabilizes the pelvis and abducts the affected side (A), extends (B), then adducts the hip (C), and finishes the test with the patient rest in the starting position (D).

NSAIDs alone have not been found to be effective in providing symptom relief. However, several studies have shown that NSAIDs, in association with other nonsurgical modalities such as rehabilitation and activity modification may be beneficial [3].

6.1.3 Rehabilitation

Physical therapy is an important part of the nonsurgical management of ITBS.

Typical rehabilitation programs consist of specific stretching exercises focused on the ITB, tensor fascia latae, and gluteus medius [22] (Fig. 4.7).

Manual therapy that consists in soft tissue and medial patellar mobilizations may also contribute to lengthening the ITB.

Active release soft-tissue mobilization techniques have gained popularity but study results are not conclusive.

Additionally, the patient can use a foam roller as a myofascial release tool to break up soft-tissue adhesions in the ITB (Fig. 4.8).

Once the patient can perform the stretching exercises without pain, strengthening is added to the rehabilitation program [2]. Attention is paid to proximal strengthening of the hip abductors (gluteus medius) and the core muscles to stabilize the pelvis and prevent excessive adduction of the hip (Fig. 4.9).

Modalities such as cryotherapy may also be incorporated into the physical therapy program to reduce the inflammatory component of the condition.

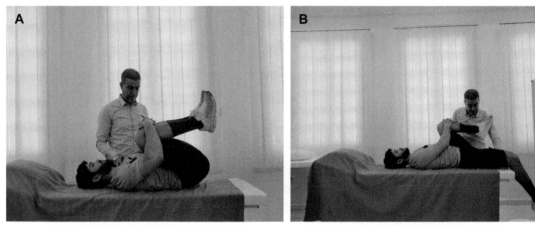

FIG. 4.6 **Pictures Illustration the Thomas Test.** The patient lies supine and holds both knees flexed to his chest (A), then he releases the affected side and the examiner verifies if complete hip extension is achieved (B).

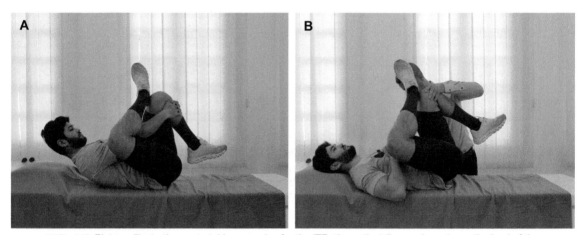

FIG. 4.7 Pictures illustrating a stretching exercise for the ITB: the patient lies supine, places the heel of the affected side on the other knee, and performs passive hip flexion of the unaffected side (A), he may be aided by the physiotherapist (B).

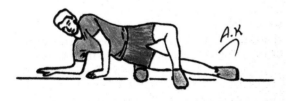

FIG. 4.8 Drawing illustrating the use of a foam roller to break up adhesions in the ITB. The patient lies sideways and performs proximodistal movements on the foam roller.

Education about proper running form and running progression are important in getting athletes back to their goals. Biomechanical studies have shown that faster-paced running is less likely to aggravate ITB. Therefore, faster strides are initially recommended over slow jogging [23].

6.2 Procedures

Corticosteroid injections next to the lateral femoral epicondyle are recommended for patients with persistent pain and swelling [24] (Fig. 4.10).

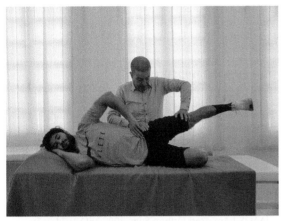

FIG. 4.9 Picture showing a gluteus medialis strengthening technique consisting in resisted lateral leg raise. The patient lies on his side and is instructed to rise the leg with the hip and knee extended, while the physiotherapist applies resistance to this movement.

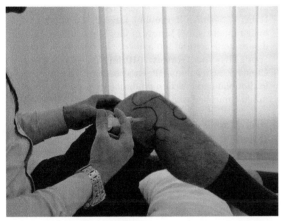

FIG. 4.10 Picture illustrating the needle placement for corticosteroids injection next to the lateral femoral condyle to treat ITBS.

A mixture of anesthetic (e.g., 1 mL of 1% lidocaine) and long-acting steroid (e.g., 1 mL of betamethasone) is used. This procedure has been used in runners with acute ITBS with good results [25].

Steroid injections should be repeated only if adequate relief is obtained after the initial injection.

6.2.1 Foot orthoses

An orthosis used to raise the heel in runners may decrease the flexion angle of the knee at foot strike and may decrease symptoms [10].

6.3 Surgical Management

Most patients have symptomatic relief without surgery within 6–8 weeks and are able to return to their athletic activities with no long-term consequences [2], but refractory cases exist.

Surgical intervention is typically reserved for patients who continue to be symptomatic and functionally limited for more than 6 months despite an adequate treatment with oral NSAIDs, physical therapy, and a corticosteroid injection.

One surgical treatment option is the percutaneous release of the ITB under local anesthesia [12].

Open surgical release involves excising a portion of the ITB directly over the lateral epicondyle.

ITB Z-lengthening is also an option. Two transverse incisions are made halfway across its width at the proximal and distal extents of the area to be lengthened.

An open ITB bursectomy has also been described to manage recalcitrant ITBS.

The arthroscopic management of refractory ITBS with liberation and resection of the lateral synovial recess appears to be promising as a minimally invasive technique to relieve symptoms and allow successful return to play [26].

7 TAKE HOME MESSAGES

ITBS is a common overuse injury typically seen in runners, cyclists, and military recruits.

The diagnosis of this condition is mainly clinical based on specific clinical tests: Renne's test, The Noble test, The Ober test, and The Thomas test.

Affected patients report lateral knee pain associated with repetitive motion activities.

Imaging studies are reserved for recalcitrant cases to rule out other pathologic entities.

The treatment is commonly conservative. However, a surgical management is indicated in persistent or chronic cases.

REFERENCES

[1] Renne JW. The iliotibial band friction syndrome. J Bone Joint Surg Am December 1975;57(8):1110–1.

[2] Lavine R. Iliotibial band friction syndrome. Curr Rev Musculoskelet Med July 20, 2010;3(1–4):18–22.

[3] Ellis R, Hing W, Reid D. Iliotibial band friction syndrome–a systematic review. Man Ther August 2007; 12(3):200–8.

[4] Farrell KC, Reisinger KD, Tillman MD. Force and repetition in cycling: possible implications for iliotibial band friction syndrome. Knee March 2003;10(1):103–9.

[5] Tuite MJ. Imaging of triathlon injuries. Radiol Clin November 2010;48(6):1125–35.

[6] Rumball JS, Lebrun CM, Di Ciacca SR, Orlando K. Rowing injuries. Sports Med Auckl NZ 2005;35(6): 537–55.

[7] Grau S, Krauss I, Maiwald C, Axmann D, Horstmann T, Best R. Kinematic classification of iliotibial band syndrome in runners. Scand J Med Sci Sports April 2011; 21(2):184–9.

[8] Noble CA. Iliotibial band friction syndrome in runners. Am J Sports Med August 1980;8(4):232–4.

[9] Kibler WB, Medicine AOS for S, Surgeons AA of O. OKU orthopaedic knowledge update. In: Sports medicine. 4th ed., vol. 4. Rosemont, IL: American Academy of Orthopaedic Surgeons; 2009 Available from: https://trove.nla. gov.au/version/34948251.

[10] Orchard JW, Fricker PA, Abud AT, Mason BR. Biomechanics of iliotibial band friction syndrome in runners. Am J Sports Med June 1996;24(3):375–9.

[11] Khaund R, Flynn SH. Iliotibial band syndrome: a common source of knee pain. Am Fam Physician April 15, 2005;71(8):1545–50.

[12] Holmes JC, Pruitt AL, Whalen NJ. Iliotibial band syndrome in cyclists. Am J Sports Med June 1993;21(3):419–24.

[13] Fredericson M, Weir A. Practical management of iliotibial band friction syndrome in runners. Clin J Sport Med Off J Can Acad Sport Med May 2006;16(3):261–8.

[14] Muhle C, Ahn JM, Yeh L, Bergman GA, Boutin RD, Schweitzer M, et al. Iliotibial band friction syndrome: MR imaging findings in 16 patients and MR arthrographic study of six cadaveric knees. Radiology 1999;212(1):103–10.

[15] Michels F, Jambou S, Allard M, Bousquet V, Colombet P, De Lavigne C. An arthroscopic technique to treat the iliotibial band syndrome. Knee Surg Sports Traumatol Arthrosc 2009;17(3):233–6.

[16] Richards DP, Barber FA, Troop RL. Iliotibial band Z-lengthening. Arthrosc J Arthrosc Relat Surg 2003;19(3):326–9.

[17] Chang KS, Cheng YH, Wu CH, Özçakar L. Dynamic ultrasound imaging for the iliotibial band/snapping hip syndrome. Am J Phys Med Rehabil 2015;94(6): e55–6.

[18] Lewis CL. Extra-articular snapping hip: a literature review. Sport Health 2010;2(3):186–90.

[19] Gyaran IA, Spiezia F, Hudson Z, Maffulli N. Sonographic measurement of iliotibial band thickness: an observational study in healthy adult volunteers. Knee Surg Sports Traumatol Arthrosc 2011;19(3):458–61.

[20] Devan MR, Pescatello LS, Faghri P, Anderson J. A prospective study of overuse knee injuries among female athletes with muscle imbalances and structural abnormalities. J Athl Train 2004;39(3):263.

[21] Wanich T, Hodgkins C, Columbier JA, Muraski E, Kennedy JG. Cycling injuries of the lower extremity. JAAOS-J Am Acad Orthop Surg. 2007;15(12):748–56.

[22] Fredericson M, White JJ, Macmahon JM, Andriacchi TP. Quantitative analysis of the relative effectiveness of 3 iliotibial band stretches. Arch Phys Med Rehabil May 2002; 83(5):589–92.

[23] Fredericson M, Wolf C. Iliotibial band syndrome in runners: innovations in treatment. Sports Med Auckl NZ 2005;35(5):451–9.

[24] Ferber R, Noehren B, Hamill J, Davis IS. Competitive female runners with a history of iliotibial band syndrome demonstrate atypical hip and knee kinematics. J Orthop Sports Phys Ther February 2010;40(2):52–8.

[25] Gunter P, Schwellnus MP. Local corticosteroid injection in iliotibial band friction syndrome in runners: a randomised controlled trial. Br J Sports Med June 2004;38(3): 269–72. discussion 272.

[26] Hariri S, Savidge ET, Reinold MM, Zachazewski J, Gill TJ. Treatment of recalcitrant iliotibial band friction syndrome with open iliotibial band bursectomy: indications, technique, and clinical outcomes. Am J Sports Med July 2009;37(7):1417–24.

CHAPTER 5

Pes Anserinus Syndrome

1 BACKGROUND

The distal insertion of the sartorius, gracilis, and semitendinosus tendons forms a structure that resembles the goose's foot. Therefore, this structure has been called "goose foot" (pes anserinus in Latin).

These muscles are primarily flexors of the knee and accessory internal rotators. They have a protecting role against external rotation and valgus stress on the knee [1]. The anserine bursa is one of 11 bursae found around the knee, located immediately below the pes anserinus.

The first description of changes in this region in the literature dates back to 1937 when Moschcowitz reported knee pain almost exclusively in women, present when going downstairs or upstairs, when rising from a chair, or having difficulty when flexing the knee [2].

The distinction between anserine bursitis and tendinitis is difficult clinically due to the proximity of the tissues. However, this distinction is not important because treatment is the same for both conditions.

This condition has been especially observed in long-distance runners [3]. Etiology includes microtrauma, retraction of posterior thigh muscles, bone exostosis, irritation of the suprapatellar plica, medial meniscus lesions, flat foot, genu valgum, local infection, and foreign body reaction [4].

Epidemiological studies suggest that anserine tendinopathy is also common in overweight females with osteoarthritis of the knees [1,5]. Diabetes mellitus has been identified in a large proportion of patients with pes anserinus [6]. Cases of chronic bursitis have been documented in patients with rheumatoid arthritis and knee osteoarthritis [7,8].

Although the majority of authors call this condition "anserine bursitis" the structure responsible for the symptoms remains unidentified in most cases [5].

The diagnosis is frequently established based on typical patient history and clinical findings, but in some cases, imaging modalities may be required.

Treatment is mainly conservative for this condition.

2 SYNONYMS

Anserine bursitis.
  Goose foot tendinopathy.

3 CLINICAL STUDY

3.1 Symptoms

The patient's history is usually typical and characterized by pain in the medial aspect of the knee, approximately 5 cm below the medial joint line. Signs of degenerative joint disease may be present. This pain may be aggravated when going upstairs or downstairs. However, it can be present in the posteromedial region or in the middle of the knee, without edema, making the differential diagnosis with meniscal lesion a challenge.

Criteria for the diagnosis of this condition was described in 1985 by Larson and Baum [7]. These criteria include:
- Pain in the anteromedial region of the knee, especially when going upstairs or downstairs.
- Morning pain and rigidity for more than 1 h.
- Nocturnal pain.
- Difficulty rising from a chair or getting out of the car.

3.2 Physical Examination

Tenderness and swelling may be present on palpation of the medial aspect of the knee.

Resisted contraction and stretching of the affected muscles usually reproduce the patient's pain.

The knee range of motion (ROM) is usually not affected.

4 DIFFERENTIAL DIAGNOSIS

Several etiologies of medial knee pain should be considered in the differential diagnosis.

4.1 L3-L4 Radiculopathy

In this case, an associated lumbar pain is present and knee pain is not aggravated on digital pressure of the anserine region.

4.2 Meniscal Cyst

The patient presents with pain, blocked movement, and a palpable mass in the articular line.

4.3 Synovial Osteochondromatosis

The patient usually presents with arthralgia, a palpable mass, and restriction of movement.

Knee Pain in Sports Medicine. https://doi.org/10.1016/B978-0-323-88069-5.00002-0

4.4 Malignant Tumors

These tumors usually have a solid component which allows to make the differential diagnosis.

5 IMAGING

5.1 Standard X-rays

They are usually normal, but can also show bony exostosis or signs of osteoarthritis of the medial compartment (Fig. 5.1).

5.2 Ultrasound

Studies have demonstrated that only a minority of patients with pes anserinus syndrome have specific ultrasound (US) changes.

A marked tendinous thickening and loss of normal fibrillar structure of the symptomatic side compared to the asymptomatic one can be observed. Fluid collection in the symptomatic anserine bursa area may also be noticed.

5.3 CT Scan

Computed tomography (CT) scan can show a well-defined cystic image of low attenuation immediately

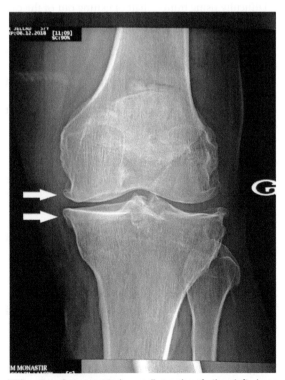

FIG. 5.1 Anteroposterior radiograph of the left knee showing medial compartment osteoarthritis with osteophytes (*arrows*).

below the pes anserinus in relation to a bursitis. It should be noted that the distension of the anserine bursa is not always synonymous of bursitis and the observed signs could be related to a case of tendinitis or fasciitis of the pes anserinus [9].

5.4 Magnetic Resonance Imaging

Magnetic resonance imaging (MRI) may be useful in the diagnosis of acute anserine bursitis when fluid accumulation and synovial proliferation are observed [10]. It is also useful in the evaluation of uncertain masses in the medial region of the knee [11] (Figs. 5.2 and 5.3).

Axial incidence is considered essential to differentiate the anserine bursa from other medial knee fluid collections. Confusion on imaging exams can be caused by cystic disorders of the knee including popliteal cyst, semimembranosus bursitis, and meniscal cyst (Fig. 5.4).

Identifying the presence of fluid in the anserine bursa associated with the classical clinical symptoms allows for a certain diagnosis [12].

6 TREATMENT

6.1 Conservative Management

6.1.1 Activity modification

The initial treatment should include resting the affected knee to avoid the progression of the pathology.

The use of a pillow between the thighs at night can be necessary to avoid worsening pain by friction between the medial aspects of the knees.

Weight loss is mandatory in obese patients.

6.1.2 Medical treatment

For acute cases, antiinflammatory drugs such as nonsteroidal antiinflammatory drugs (NSAIDs) and analgesics such as paracetamol can provide pain relief and are indicated in association with other modalities of conservative management.

6.1.3 Rehabilitation

Physical agents may have a role in the treatment of this disorder. US has been recognized to be effective in reducing inflammation in anserine tendinopathy [8]. Transcutaneous electrical nerve stimulation is another physical modality that may be used. It has been successfully used in other types of bursitis, but has not been documented specifically in this condition.

Rehabilitation programs should include stretching exercises of muscles with tendons that comprise the pes anserinus and strengthening of hip adductors and

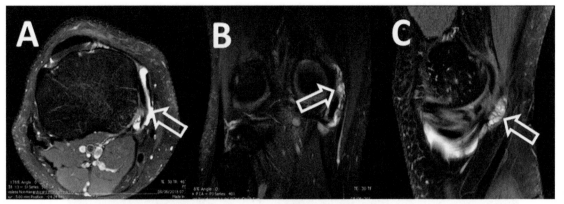

FIG. 5.2 T2-weighted MRI sequences of the knee illustrating a hyperintense signal (*arrows*) in axial (A), coronal (B), and sagittal (C) sections in relation to an acute anserine bursitis.

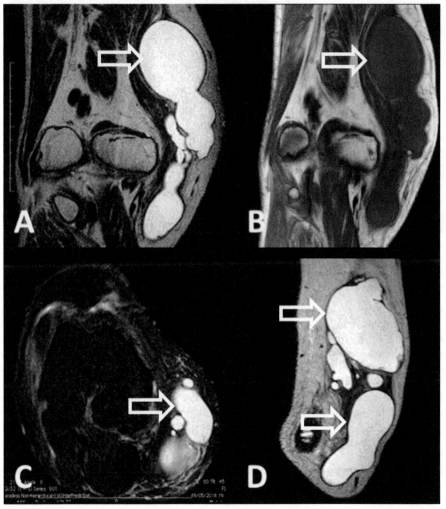

FIG. 5.3 Knee MRI sequences in coronal (A and B), axial (C), and sagittal (D) views illustrating a large anserine bursitis (*arrows*).

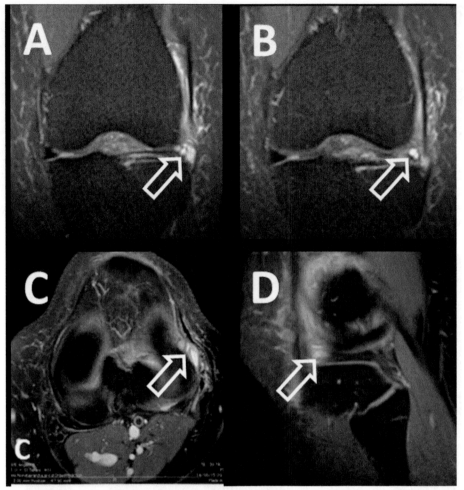

FIG. 5.4 MRI of the left knee without Gadolinium injection, in coronal (A and B), axial (C), and sagittal (D) DP FAT SAT sections illustrating lateral cystic formation at the expense of the middle segment of the lateral meniscus in relation to a meniscal cyst (*arrows*).

quadriceps, especially in the last 30° of knee extension, focusing on the vastus medialis muscle.

For cases related to muscle inflexibility and muscles/tendons retraction, stretching can provide an important reduction in the tension on the anserine bursa. Treatment of occasional associated conditions, such as deviated knee and flat feet, and control of diabetes should be considered to optimize the rehabilitation treatment results.

6.2 Procedures

In case of a documented bursitis, the injection of a local anesthetic associated with corticosteroids in the bursa is recommended. Methylprednisolone at the dose of 20–40 mg of can be injected as well as triamcinolone,

or betamethasone [13,14]. Special care should be taken to avoid injecting the substance in the tendons of the pes anserinus.

No more than three infiltrations should be done over a one-year period. The time between infiltrations should be greater than one month [14].

Patients who do not show any response to an initial infiltration rarely respond to repeated infiltrations.

Associating an injection in the knee joint can be beneficial in refractory cases [13].

The risk of complications include atrophy of the subcutaneous tissue, skin depigmentation, and rupture of the tendon [15]. Patients should be informed about discomfort or pain after the injection, which is seen in 30% of the patients, and 10% are at risk of developing a local reaction to the corticosteroid. These side effects can be managed with local ice therapy and analgesics [16].

6.3 Surgical Treatment

Surgery is indicated in case of failure of the conservative treatment especially when a bursitis is present.

An incision followed by drainage of the distended bursa can provide immediate improvement of symptoms [17].

The complete removal of the bursa is indicated when the lesion is large in size [4]. Associated bone exostosis should be removed to avoid the recurrence of symptoms.

7 TAKE HOME MESSAGES

Pes anserinus syndrome is a frequent etiology of microtraumatic medial knee pain.

The diagnosis of this condition is mainly clinical, based on typical patient history and clinical examination findings. The diagnostic criteria include:
- Pain in the anteromedial region of the knee, especially going upstairs or downstairs.
- Morning pain and rigidity for more than one hour.
- Nocturnal pain.
- Difficulty rising from a chair or getting out of the car.

Imaging techniques such as MRI and US are useful in nontypical cases.

Conservative management consists of relative rest, physical therapy, and corticosteroids injections.

Surgery is indicated in cases of failure of the conservative treatment.

REFERENCES

[1] Alvarez-Nemegyei J, Canoso JJ. Evidence-based soft tissue rheumatology IV: anserine bursitis. J Clin Rheumatol Pract Rep Rheum Musculoskelet Dis August 2004;10(4): 205—6.

[2] Moschcowitz E. Bursitis of sartorius bursa: an undescribed malady simulating chronic arthritis. J Am Med Assoc October 23, 1937;109(17). 1362—1362.

[3] Safran M, Zachazewski JE, Stone DA. Instructions for sports medicine patients. Elsevier Health Sciences; 2011.

[4] Huang TW, Wang CJ, Huang SC. Polyethylene-induced pes anserinus bursitis mimicking an infected total knee arthroplasty: a case report and review of the literature. J Arthroplasty April 1, 2003;18(3):383—6.

[5] Gnanadesigan N, Smith RL. Knee pain: osteoarthritis or anserine bursitis? J Am Med Dir Assoc June 2003;4(3): 164—6.

[6] Cohen SE, Mahul O, Meir R, Rubinow A. Anserine bursitis and non-insulin dependent diabetes mellitus. J Rheumatol November 1997;24(11):2162—5.

[7] Larsson LG, Baum J. The syndrome of anserina bursitis: an overlooked diagnosis. Arthritis Rheum September 1985;28(9):1062—5.

[8] Brooker MI, Mongan ES. Anserina bursitis—a treatable cause of knee pain in patients with degenerative arthritis. Calif Med July 1973;119(1):8—10.

[9] Hall FM, Joffe N. CT imaging of the anserine bursa. AJR Am J Roentgenol May 1988;150(5):1107—8.

[10] Forbes JR, Helms CA, Janzen DL. Acute pes anserine bursitis: MR imaging. Radiology February 1995;194(2): 525—7.

[11] Muchnick J, Sundaram M. Radiologic case study. Pes anserine bursitis. Orthopedics November 1997;20(11). 1100; 1092—1094.

[12] Rennie WJ, Saifuddin A. Pes anserine bursitis: incidence in symptomatic knees and clinical presentation. Skeletal Radiol July 2005;34(7):395—8.

[13] Abeles M. Osteoarthritis of the knee-anserine bursitis as an extra-articular cause of pain. In: Clinical research. THOROFARE, NJ: SLACK INC 6900 GROVE RD; 1983. p. 08086. A447—A447.

[14] O'donoghue DH. Treatment of injuries to athletes. WB Saunders Company; 1984.

[15] Saunders S, Longworth S. Injection techniques in orthopaedic and sports medicine: a practical manual for doctors and physiotherapists. Elsevier Health Sciences; 2006.

[16] Anderson BC. Office orthopedics for primary care: diagnosis and treatment (ed 2). J Muscoskel Med 1999; 16(7). 415—415.

[17] Zeiss J, Coombs RJ, Booth JR, Saddemi SR. Chronic bursitis presenting as a mass in the pes anserine bursa: MR diagnosis. J Comput Assist Tomogr 1993;17(1): 137—40.

CHAPTER 6

Biceps Femoris Tendinopathy

1 BACKGROUND

Biceps femoris (BF) muscle injuries are common sports injuries that can affect both recreational and elite athletes [1].

These injuries have gained considerable attention because of the time lost from sports and the burden on both athletes and their teams. Although fairly common, these types of injuries are considered a difficult entity to treat. The first step in treating these injuries is an accurate and rapid diagnosis.

The majority of these injuries are limited to tendon strains, but if diagnosis is not made early, the treatment results and the outcome will be badly affected [2]. These injuries have a tendency to recur, especially in elite athletes, and some patients may develop chronic symptoms.

The exact rate of BF injuries varies as a result of different definitions of what qualifies as an injury and the diversity of populations studied [3]. In general, the prevalence of all hamstring injuries ranges from 8% to 25% of all athletes' injuries [3,4]. Epidemiological data regarding BF injuries are currently lacking.

The prevalence of BF tendinopathy is higher in sports associated with running and fast acceleration which result in increased stress on the BF muscle-tendon junction unit. These injuries are frequently seen in sports such as soccer, American football, gymnastics, and water skiing [5]. Tendon strains are considered the most common form of injury, while complete ruptures occur less frequently [6].

Multiple risk factors have been described [3]. Modifiable factors include muscular fatigue, low muscular strength, lack of warm-up, higher level of competition, and low hamstring to quadriceps strength ratio. Non-modifiable factors include age, previous injury, and black race [7]. A previous hamstring injury is considered the greatest risk factor and is associated with an increase in the rate of reinjury [8]. Age was reported to be an important independent predictor of hamstring injury [9]. In elite athletes, speed and kicking positions have been found to increase the risk of injury [10].

Distal BF tendon injuries are less frequent than proximal ones, even though they share the same mechanism, which includes both eccentric muscular contraction during the stance phase of running and overstretching the leg [10].

2 SYNONYMS

BF Strain.
  BF partial rupture.
  BF tendinosis

3 CLINICAL STUDY

3.1 Symptoms

History is characterized by the absence of acute trauma. Usually there is an insidious onset of posterior knee pain, and a difficulty in weight-bearing activities. Patients may rarely have difficulty sitting as a result of pain. In the early phase of the injury, walking can be hard and running is often impossible [11]. Some patients can also present with neuropathic pain in the posterior thigh. This clinical presentation called gluteal sciatica is related to compression of the sciatic nerve resulting from scarring and typically involves mainly the posterior cutaneous branch of the sciatic nerve (Fig. 6.1).

Patients often report weakness in knee flexion associated with pain and stiffness. Depending on the severity of the condition, patients may have a loss of active flexion and in some cases may have difficulty with active extension. In addition, cramps and spasms in the posterior aspect of the thigh are possible.

Patients with chronic injuries usually present with profound weakness rather than pain. In addition, gluteal sciatica symptoms are more frequent in the chronic phase due to excessive scarring in the area of injury and subsequent nerve irritation [11].

3.2 Physical Examination

Identifying a BF injury during physical examination can be difficult because of the deep location of the muscle within the thigh. However, there are some signs that may guide the examiner toward the diagnosis. In case of a rupture, a palpable defect can be occasionally felt along the course of the tendon.

Knee Pain in Sports Medicine. https://doi.org/10.1016/B978-0-323-88069-5.00016-0

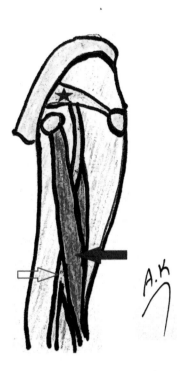

FIG. 6.1 Anatomic representation showing the relation between sciatic nerve (empty *arrow*) the long head of the BF muscle (full *arrow*) and piriformis muscle (star).

An important part of the physical examination is testing knee range of motion (ROM) and the strength of the affected muscle and comparing these findings with those on the contralateral side.

Ideally, the patient should be lying prone with the hip positioned in 0 degree of extension. Knee flexion is then examined with resistance applied at the heel with the knee in 15 degrees and 90 degrees of flexion (Fig. 6.2).

Pain provoked by the examination or weakness is considered a positive finding [12].

Hip flexion and knee extension should be examined to test BF flexibility which can be limited by pain [1] (Fig. 6.3).

4 DIFFERENTIAL DIAGNOSIS

4.1 Lateral Osteoarthritis of the Knee or Osteochondral Defects

Pain is rather felt as intraarticular and patients present with a swelling of variable amounts.

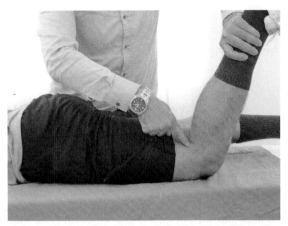

FIG. 6.2 Picture illustrating the palpation of the BF tendon: the patient tries to flex his knee, while the examiner opposes this movement and exerts an external tibial rotation.

4.2 Injury to the Lateral Collateral Ligament or Posterolateral Corner of the Knee

A history of acute trauma is usually found and signs of instability may be present.

4.3 Lateral Meniscal Tears

Locking sensations are frequently present and meniscal tests are positive.

4.4 Iliotibial Band Syndrome

Lateral knee pain and a snapping sensation of the knee in runners and cyclists is suggestive of this syndrome. Specific clinical tests allow to confirm the diagnosis.

5 IMAGING

5.1 Standard X-rays

All young athletes complaining from an acute onset of pain should be evaluated with radiographs to identify avulsion fractures [5].

Other findings include soft tissue swelling, but it is usually difficult to appreciate radiographically. At the chronic stage, calcifications may appear in the tendon area, but they are quite uncommon.

5.2 Ultrasound

Ultrasound (US) has been reported to be an excellent tool for diagnosing BF tendinopathy.

It is easily accessible and is less expensive than magnetic resonance imaging (MRI). However, it is highly operator-dependent, and diagnosing small injuries is sometimes challenging.

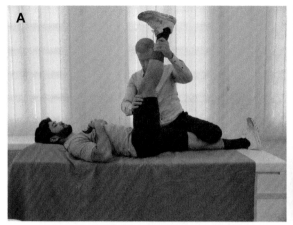 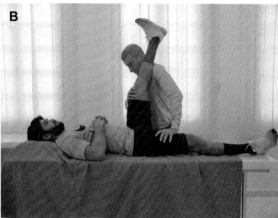

FIG. 6.3 Pictures (A) and (B) illustrating two techniques for testing hamstring extensibility. The patient lies supine, the examiner flexes the hip and attempts to extend the knee. Hamstring inflexibility is marked by lack of complete knee extension.

Furthermore, in some cases, it can be difficult to differentiate scar tissue of an old injury from an acute injury [13].

5.3 CT Scan

Computed tomography (CT) scan has been used by some authors to evaluate BF tendinopathies in their acute stages. In fact, it allowed to accurately localize and determine the extent of the lesions. The affected area appeared as a zone of low density suggesting the presence of edema [14].

5.4 Magnetic Resonance Imaging

MRI is considered as the standard modality for the diagnosis of distal BF injuries [15]. This is particularly true in cases of recurrent injuries [13].

It is also crucial for determining the extent of the injury and differentiating between partial and complete tears and the amount of retraction in case of tendon rupture [13,15].

Findings include high signal intensity areas in acute injuries on T2-weighted sequences as a result of surrounding edema.

The same areas appear as intermediate signal zones on T1-weighted sequences [16]. MRI aspects of chronic lesions are very diverse, but it is important to mention that axial sequences are the most helpful in their diagnosis.

MRI findings have also been shown to be helpful in predicting the duration of the postinjury rehabilitation period by correlation to the length and cross-sectional area of the injury [16]. Cohen et al. found that MRI

predictors for increased time away from sports included muscle retraction, and a long high signal on sagittal plane on T2-weighted sequences [17].

6 TREATMENT

6.1 Conservative Treatment

RICE protocol should be followed in the initial management of this tendinopathy.

6.1.1 Activity modification

The use of compressive clothing, incorporation of warm-up and cool-down exercises before and after sports activities, and joint proprioception training have been reported as factors that can decrease the risk of BF tendinopathy and their recurrence [18].

6.1.2 Medical treatment

Nonsteroidal antiinflammatory drugs (NSAIDs) have been suggested as an option for reducing the inflammation and pain perception, but the effect of such drugs on reducing the intensity of symptomatic aspects of BF muscle injuries has not been studied [19].

6.1.3 Rehabilitation

The main purpose of any rehabilitation program included in the operative or nonoperative treatment of BF injury is to restore the patient's functional capacities.

Multiple studies have shown the effectiveness of eccentric strengthening in reducing the risk of sustaining this type of injury, both as a preventive measure

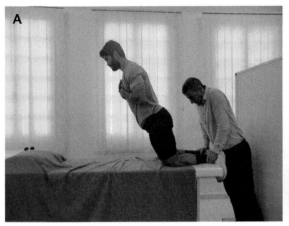

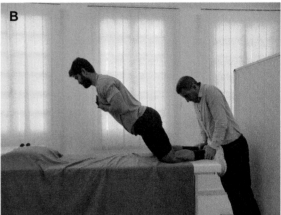

FIG. 6.4 Pictures illustrating the Nordic hamstring curls. While the athlete is kneeling on the table, the physiotherapist stabilizes the athlete's shins (A) while he lowers his torso slowly using an eccentric contraction of hamstring muscles (B).

and in patients with established strains, especially when preceded by an adequate duration of warm-up stretching [4].

Exercises directed at trunk stabilization and core strengthening have also been shown to reduce the risk of injuries in this muscle (134). Neuromuscular control and eccentric strengthening exercises, such as Nordic hamstring exercises are recommended in rehabilitation programs for patients with acute injuries [4] (Fig. 6.4).

The theory is that stretching and strengthening in the rehabilitation process of acute BF tendinopathy can help to remodel and align collagen fibers in the tendon [20]. Some authors have advanced that lumbopelvic neuromuscular control, including anterior and posterior pelvic tilt, is very important for optimizing hamstring muscle function and therefore have suggested the implementation of a progressive agility and trunk stabilization rehabilitation program [21] (Fig. 6.5).

Sherry and Best showed that individuals with an acute hamstring injury who were managed with this kind of program had a lower reinjury rate than patients who were managed with a progressive stretching and strengthening program alone [20].

The patients should be assessed before returning to sports, but there is no good evidence in the literature for a functional test that can predict or guide the timing of returning to sports with a low reinjury rate. General criteria that have been mentioned in the literature for the return to play include full strength and ROM without pain, a symmetrical knee flexion angle, and comfortable replication of sport-specific movements at the competition level [22].

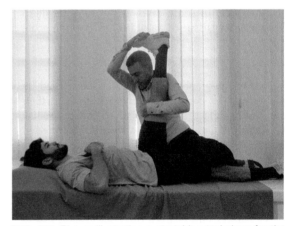

FIG. 6.5 Picture illustrating a stretching technique for the posterior chain muscles of the lower limbs including hamstrings.

Treatment modalities such as US stimulation, cold and heat pads, and massage have been described for the treatment of hamstring injuries with moderate validity [23].

6.2 Procedures

Peritendinous corticosteroid injections have been found to accelerate the return to the preinjury level of competition capacities, but some studies have shown unfavorable effects on the healing process of the injured muscle, and this method remains controversial [22].

Recent attention has been directed toward the use of platelet-rich plasma (PRP) injections for the treatment of BF tendinopathy, with promising results in some studies [23].

Recommendations also point to the avoidance of complete immobilization of the injured limb to avoid atrophy of the muscle [19].

6.3 Surgical Treatment

Surgical treatment should be reserved for cases of tendon rupture and recalcinent tendinopathy.

Many techniques have been described, but there is no clear consensus regarding the operative treatment of BF muscle injuries [3].

There is a paucity of literature on the surgical treatment of chronic BF tendinopathies. In a study, tendon repair after excision of scar tissue was performed and patients had good to excellent results and managed to return to their previous level of sports activity [3].

7 TAKE HOME MESSAGES

BF tendinopathies are common sports injuries and a leading cause of time away from sports.

Previous hamstring injury and age are considered the most important risk factors for these injuries in both elite and recreational athletes.

The diagnosis will be made based on an accurate patient history (especially an insidious onset of posterior knee pain) and a thorough physical examination (pain on palpation and muscle resisted contraction and stretching).

MRI and US are the modalities of choice for the diagnosis of this injury. MRI has a prognostic value by correlation to the length and cross-sectional area of the injury.

Rehabilitation is the cornerstone of conservative treatment and should concentrate on both eccentric strengthening and proprioceptive and core exercises.

Complete BF tendon rupture should be treated surgically.

REFERENCES

[1] Heiderscheit BC, Sherry MA, Silder A, Chumanov ES, Thelen DG. Hamstring strain injuries: recommendations for diagnosis, rehabilitation, and injury prevention. J Orthop Sports Phys Ther 2010;40(2):67–81.

[2] Folsom GJ, Larson CM. Surgical treatment of acute versus chronic complete proximal hamstring ruptures: results of a new allograft technique for chronic reconstructions. Am J Sports Med 2008;36(1):104–9.

[3] Copland ST, Tipton JS, Fields KB. Evidence-based treatment of hamstring tears. Curr Sports Med Rep 2009; 8(6):308–14.

[4] Askling C, Karlsson J, Thorstensson A. Hamstring injury occurrence in elite soccer players after preseason strength training with eccentric overload. Scand J Med Sci Sports 2003;13(4):244–50.

[5] Clanton TO, Coupe KJ. Hamstring strains in athletes: diagnosis and treatment. JAAOS-J Am Acad Orthop Surg. 1998;6(4):237–48.

[6] Cohen SE, Mahul O, Meir R, Rubinow A. Anserine bursitis and non-insulin dependent diabetes mellitus. J Rheumatol November 1997;24(11):2162–5.

[7] Brooks JH, Fuller CW, Kemp SP, Reddin DB. Incidence, risk, and prevention of hamstring muscle injuries in professional rugby union. Am J Sports Med 2006;34(8): 1297–306.

[8] Mendiguchia J, Alentorn-Geli E, Brughelli M. Hamstring strain injuries: are we heading in the right direction. BMJ Publishing Group Ltd and British Association of Sport and Exercise Medicine; 2012.

[9] Gabbe BJ, Bennell KL, Finch CF, Wajswelner H, Orchard JW. Predictors of hamstring injury at the elite level of Australian football. Scand J Med Sci Sports 2006;16(1):7–13.

[10] Lempainen L, Banke IJ, Johansson K, Brucker PU, Sarimo J, Orava S, et al. Clinical principles in the management of hamstring injuries. Knee Surg Sports Traumatol Arthrosc 2015;23(8):2449–56.

[11] Price RJ, Hawkins RD, Hulse MA. The football association medical research programme: an audit of injuries in academy youth football. Change 2002;2(4):6.

[12] Kujala UM, Orava S, Järvinen M. Hamstring injuries. Sports Med 1997;23(6):397–404.

[13] Schneider-Kolsky ME, Hoving JL, Warren P, Connell DA. A comparison between clinical assessment and magnetic resonance imaging of acute hamstring injuries. Am J Sports Med 2006;34(6):1008–15.

[14] Connell DA, Schneider-Kolsky ME, Hoving JL, Malara F, Buchbinder R, Koulouris G, et al. Longitudinal study comparing sonographic and MRI assessments of acute and healing hamstring injuries. Am J Roentgenol 2004; 183(4):975–84.

[15] Cohen S, Bradley J. Acute proximal hamstring rupture. JAAOS-J Am Acad Orthop Surg. 2007;15(6):350–5.

[16] Brandser EA, El-Khoury GY, Kathol MH, Callaghan JJ, Tearse DS. Hamstring injuries: radiographic, conventional tomography, CT, and MR imaging characteristics. Radiology 1995;197(1):257–62.

[17] Koulouris G, Connell DA, Brukner P, Schneider-Kolsky M. Magnetic resonance imaging parameters for assessing risk of recurrent hamstring injuries in elite athletes. Am J Sports Med 2007;35(9):1500–6.

[18] Dawson WJ, Petersen J, Holmich P. Evidence based prevention of hamstring injury in sport. Med Probl Perform Art 2006;21(4):191–2.

[19] Reynolds JF, Noakes TD, Schwellnus MP, Windt A, Bowerbank P. Non-steroidal antiinflammatory drugs fail to enhance healing of acute hamstring injuries treated with physiotherapy. S Afr Med J January 1, 1995;85(6).

Available from: https://www.ajol.info/index.php/samj/article/view/156043.

[20] Worrell TW. Factors associated with hamstring injuries. Sports Med 1994;17(5):338−45.

[21] Bennell K, Tully E, Harvey N. Does the toe-touch test predict hamstring injury in Australian Rules footballers? Aust J Physiother 1999;45(2):103−9.

[22] Schmitt B, Tim T, McHugh M. Hamstring injury rehabilitation and prevention of reinjury using lengthened state eccentric training: a new concept. Int J Sports Phys Ther June 2012;7(3):333−41.

[23] Petersen J, Hölmich P. Evidence based prevention of hamstring injuries in sport. Br J Sports Med June 1, 2005;39(6):319−23.

CHAPTER 7

Popliteus Tendinopathy

1 BACKGROUND

Although tendinopathy popliteus is a common injury in athletes, it is often misdiagnosed because of the anatomical and biomechanical particularities of the popliteus muscle.

Overuse of the muscle-tendon junction unit has been incriminated in the pathogenesis of the popliteus tendinopathy. It usually occurs in sportsmen who run or train on hills or irregular surfaces [1]. Athletes with a history of other knee injuries are also more likely to develop popliteus tendinopathy. This condition is relatively rare in the general population of nonathletes without a history of knee trauma [2,3].

Anatomically, the popliteus muscle is a small muscle located on the posterolateral corner of the knee. It has three origins: the lateral femoral condyle, the fibular head, and the lateral meniscus.

Biomechanically, this muscle performs tibial internal rotation during walking especially during the swing phase (open chain), also called endorotation of the lower leg. The most important role of the popliteus is to provide advancing stabilization of the knee and the stabilization of the lateral meniscus during knee flexion. It is considered as a flexion starter as it allows the knee to be flexed from full extension. Due to this function, the popliteus muscle is often seen as the key to unlock the knee [2,3]. The third function prevents forward displacement of the femur on the tibia and limits knee valgus when the foot is fixed to the ground (closed chain) [4]. The fourth function is to tighten the posterior capsule and help the anatomically weak capsular-ligamentous elements of the posterolateral side of the knee [4].

Several risk factors for popliteus tendinopathy have been found. These include downhill running, pace lengthening, increased distance, and over pronation of the foot or the use of bad footwear. Downhill running has been reported to be the predominant cause of this injury [1].

Clinically, this condition is characterized by pain localized to the posterolateral aspect of the knee that appears on weight-bearing activities requiring knee flexion. Specific clinical tests are needed for the diagnosis.

Clinical findings are not always typical, and in these cases, clinicians may resort to ultrasound (US) and magnetic resonance imaging (MRI) which are of great interest in diagnosing acute popliteus tendinopathy.

Surgery is an effective treatment that should be reserved for patients in which conventional therapy has failed.

2 SYNONYMS

Popliteus tendinitis.

Popliteus tendon tenosynovitis.

3 CLINICAL STUDY

3.1 Symptoms

Popliteus tendinopathy is often diagnosed in professional runners and triathletes [5]. It is uncommon in a nonathletic person without a history of knee trauma [3].

The characteristic symptom for this condition is pain localized in the posterolateral aspect of the knee that appears in the early degrees of knee flexion on weight bearing activities [6].

If the patient continues his physical activities, pain will get worse impairing activities that require knee flexion [3].

Walking, running, and going up stairs can be impaired especially in the acute stages of the injury [7]. Downhill running or walking can exacerbate symptoms by causing increased stress on the popliteus muscle-tendon unit, since this activity requires a deceleration in which the popliteus muscle is involved [8].

3.2 Physical Examination

During examination, tenderness on palpation of the posterolateral side of the lateral femoral epicondyle is found in popliteus tendinitis [9]. This pain can be associated with inflammatory signs such as localized swelling, redness, and marked tenderness at the insertion of the popliteus tendon [10]. A crepitation sound is also frequently heard when the tendon is moved [9] (Fig. 7.1).

Knee Pain in Sports Medicine. https://doi.org/10.1016/B978-0-323-88069-5.00010-X

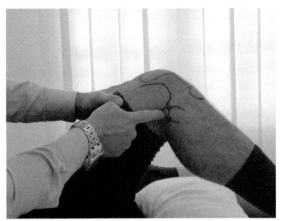

FIG. 7.1 Picture demonstrating the palpation site for the popliteus tendon: area between the lateral collateral ligament of the knee, the lateral femoral condyle, and the BF muscle tendon.

When evaluating range of motion (ROM), the knee cannot be fully extended because of the muscle tightness. while knee flexion remains normal [10]. Both knees should be examined while paying attention for asymmetry.

To test the popliteus tendon, the patient is asked to sit in "a 4 figure" position with the affected side crossed over the healthy side, the hip flexed, abducted, and externally rotated, and the knee flexed, while the therapist palpates the posterolateral corner looking for tenderness [2].

To test the popliteus muscle in closed chain, the patient stands on both feet with the knees flexed at 30 degrees. The examiner applies a valgus stress on the affected knee, while the patient opposes this movement. The test is positive if it reproduces the patient's pain (Fig. 7.2).

Another test for the popliteus muscle can be performed with the patient in supine position on the table and instructed to perform foot adduction and knee flexion, while the examiner opposes this movement [5] (Fig. 7.3).

4 DIFFERENTIAL DIAGNOSIS

The differential diagnosis of popliteus tendinopathy includes:

4.1 Posterior Horn Tear of the Meniscus

Symptoms of a posterior horn medial meniscus tear include pain localized at the posterior aspect of the knee, swelling, stiffness, catching, or locking and a sensation of instability that are aggravated with deep squatting.

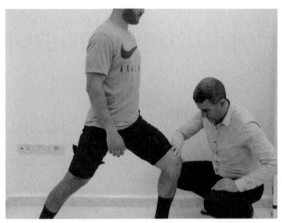

FIG. 7.2 Picture illustrating closed chain popliteus muscle testing performed in weight bearing.

4.2 Osteochondritis Dissecans

Pain and swelling of the knee often triggered by sports or physical activity are the most common initial symptoms of osteochondritis dissecans. Advanced cases may present with joint catching or locking.

4.3 Iliotibial Band Syndrome

Pain in the lateral aspect of the knee that is worsened with running downhill, cycling, or rowing is suggestive of iliotibial band syndrome (ITBS).

5 IMAGING

5.1 Standard X-rays

In some cases, conventional radiographs may show radiodensities in the region involving the popliteus tendon.

5.2 Ultrasound

The main ultrasonographic finding in patients with popliteus tendinopathy is an increase in muscle and tendon thickness.

Thickening of the popliteus muscle compared to the unaffected side can be observed on dynamic US examination during both knee flexion and extension. Increased muscle thickness during lower leg internal rotation has been reported to be present in 90% of subjects with popliteus tendinitis [11].

5.3 Magnetic Resonance Imaging

MRI is an interesting technique for detecting acute popliteus tendinopathy. Intratendinous signal alteration and abnormal thickening have been described. In fact, thickening was found in 33% in an MRI study of knees with popliteus tendinitis [11] (Fig. 7.4).

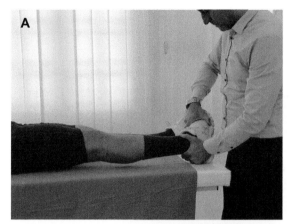

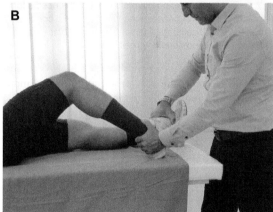

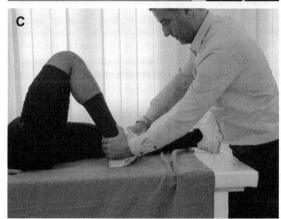

FIG. 7.3 Pictures illustrating open chain popliteus muscle testing. The patient lies supine with the knee extended and performs foot adduction (A) combined with knee flexion (B), while the examiner resists the movements to the end (C).

Excessive varus alignment of the knee was found to be a predictor of abnormal MRI findings including the increase in muscle thickness [12].

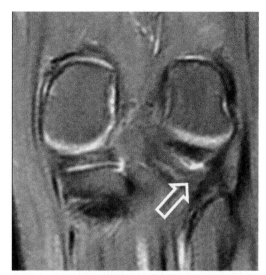

FIG. 7.4 Coronal density protonic fat saturation MRI sequences of the knee showing thickening and heterogenous signal of the popliteus tendon (*arrow*) in a patient with popliteus tendinopathy.

6 TREATMENT

6.1 Conservative Management

RICE protocol should be followed in the initial management of this tendinopathy.

6.1.1 Activity modification

Postures with extreme varus or valgus of the knee should be avoided. Patients with poor dynamic lower extremity stability should avoid fast-paced exercises [13]. Relative rest and cryotherapy may help to accelerate the healing process since they are useful to reduce pain and swelling and prevent additional damage [14].

Full immobilization must be avoided in order to prevent muscle atrophy and ROM limitation. Therefore immobilization should only be partial and activities that promote a light load on the muscle are helpful to guide the tissue healing of the tendon [15]. For example, cycling provides a good alternative exercise and helps to maintain the athlete's cardiovascular capacities.

The patients should not return to running until the knee is no longer painful, then they should limit their workouts duration and avoid downhill running for at least six weeks [16].

It is also necessary to wear correct shoe wears that prevent hyper pronation and popliteus tendinitis [17].

6.1.2 Medical treatment

Drugs such as paracetamol or ibuprofen have been proven efficient in reducing pain. If the inflammation process is active, treatment may include oral corticosteroids or nonsteroidal antiinflammatory drugs (NSAIDs). This modality of treatment should be indicated in association with other conservative approaches. It has been reported that popliteus tendinitis can be treated successfully with antiinflammatory medication for two weeks in combination with an ambulatory rehabilitation program [15].

6.1.3 Rehabilitation

Physical therapy aims to improve knee functional capacities and reduce existing limitations in ROM. The main guideline to this treatment modality should be training patients to perform their sporting activities using a painless technique.

Strengthening and stretching exercises of the popliteus muscle should be started when the pain decreases. The intensity and the duration of strengthening and stretching exercises should be increased gradually. As in other tendinopathies, the most effective form of muscle training in cases of popliteus tendinopathy remains eccentric training because it helps the collagen fibers to regenerate in the correct pattern [15]. Eccentric strengthening of the quadriceps in closed kinetic chain is helpful in reducing stress exerted on the popliteus [9].

US, shock wave therapy, and massage are physical modalities that can be used to reduce pain [18]. Performing transverse friction massage should be a part of the rehabilitation program as well since it accelerates the tendon healing process [7].

6.2 Procedures

Corticosteroid injections have been tried with satisfying results [14]. Some authors reported an immediate relief in patients injected with a combination of corticosteroids and local anesthetics [17] (Fig. 7.5).

A compression bandage or a knee brace may be very useful in reducing painful symptoms in many patients [15].

Taping of the painful knee region has been tried and studies found it to be a helpful alternative to reduce the pain [16].

6.3 Surgical Treatment

Surgery is an effective treatment that should be reserved for cases where conservative treatment has failed.

When symptoms persist for more than six months, surgery is recommended to relieve the patient [16].

Many repair and reconstruction techniques to restore the functional capacities of the popliteus tendon have been reported. These surgical modalities include primary repair, Achilles tendon allograft reconstruction [16],

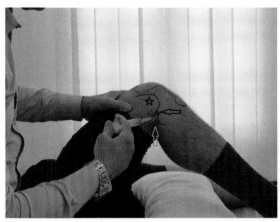

FIG. 7.5 Picture illustrating the placement of the needle for corticosteroid injection between the lateral femoral condyle (star) and the lateral collateral ligament anteriorly (*black arrow*) and the BF tendon posteriorly (*green arrow*).

augmentation using the ITB or biceps tendon, and reconstruction using patellar tendon autograft.

Following surgery, patients are restricted from performing weight-bearing and external tibial rotation activities for the first six weeks and a postoperative rehabilitation program should be planned.

7 TAKE HOME MESSAGES

Popliteus tendinopathy is a common injury in athletes, especially long-distance runners, and is prompted by training errors.

Pain localized at the posterolateral aspect of the knee is the main clinical sign. This symptom usually appears on weight bearing activities requiring knee flexion.

Clinical examination is based on open and closed chain specific muscle testing.

US and MRI are of great interest in detecting popliteus tendinopathy when the clinical presentation and physical examination findings are not typical.

Conservative management of popliteus tendinopathy is commonly sufficient to treat this condition.

Surgery is reserved for cases where conventional management has failed.

REFERENCES

[1] Safran M, Zachazewski JE, Stone DA. Instructions for sports medicine patients. Elsevier Health Sciences; 2011.
[2] Jadhav SP, More SR, Riascos RF, Lemos DF, Swischuk LE. Comprehensive review of the anatomy, function, and

imaging of the popliteus and associated pathologic conditions. Radiographics 2014;34(2):496−513.

[3] Blake SM, Treble NJ. Popliteus tendon tenosynovitis. Br J Sports Med 2005;39(12). e42−e42.

[4] LaPrade RF, Wozniczka JK, Stellmaker MP, Wijdicks CA. Analysis of the static function of the popliteus tendon and evaluation of an anatomic reconstruction: the "fifth ligament" of the knee. Am J Sports Med 2010;38(3):543−9.

[5] Olson WR, Rechkemmer L. Popliteus tendinitis. J Am Podiatr Med Assoc 1993;83(9):537−40.

[6] de Simone V, Demey G, Magnussen RA, Lustig S, Servien E, Neyret P. Iatrogenic popliteus tendon injury during total knee arthroplasty results in decreased knee function two to three years postoperatively. Int Orthop 2012;36(10):2061−5.

[7] Dutton M. Dutton's Orthopaedic examination, evaluation, and intervention. McGraw-Hill Medical; 2012.

[8] Mayfield GW. Popliteus tendon tenosynovitis. Am J Sports Med 1977;5(1):31−6.

[9] Petsche TS, Selesnick FH. Popliteus tendinitis: tips for diagnosis and management. Phys Sportsmed 2002; 30(8):27−31.

[10] Tibrewal SB. Acute calcific tendinitis of the popliteus tendon−an unusual site and clinical syndrome. Ann R Coll Surg Engl 2002;84(5):338.

[11] Soda N, Fujihashi Y, Aoki T. In vivo ultrasound imaging of the popliteus muscle: investigation of functional characteristics. J Phys Ther Sci 2016;28(3):979−82.

[12] Choi JY, Chang CB, Kim TK, Hong SH, Kang HS. Magnetic resonance imaging findings of the lateral collateral ligament and popliteus tendon in symptomatic knees without instability. Arthrosc J Arthrosc Relat Surg 2015; 31(4):665−72.

[13] Nyland J, Lachman N, Kocabey Y, Brosky J, Altun R, Caborn D. Anatomy, function, and rehabilitation of the popliteus musculotendinous complex. J Orthop Sports Phys Ther 2005;35(3):165−79.

[14] Bleakley C, McDonough S, MacAuley D. The use of ice in the treatment of acute soft-tissue injury: a systematic review of randomized controlled trials. Am J Sports Med 2004;32(1):251−61.

[15] Wilson JJ, Best TM. Common overuse tendon problems: a review and recommendations for treatment. Am Fam Physician 2005;72(5):811−8.

[16] Allardyce TJ, Scuderi GR, Insall JN. Arthroscopic treatment of popliteus tendon dysfunction following total knee arthroplasty. J Arthroplasty 1997;12(3):353−5.

[17] Clancy WG. Runners' injuries part two. Evaluation and treatment of specific injuries. Am J Sports Med 1980; 8(4):287−9.

[18] Klaiman MD, Shrader JA, Danoff JV, Hicks JE, Pesce WJ, Ferland J. Phonophoresis versus ultrasound in the treatment of common musculoskeletal conditions. Med Sci Sports Exerc 1998;30(9):1349−55.

CHAPTER 8

Ganglion Cyst and Mucoid Degeneration of the Anterior Cruciate Ligament

1 ACL GANGLION CYST

1.1 Background

Anterior cruciate ligament (ACL) ganglion cyst is a microtraumatic pathology that has been found to be associated with insidious onset of chronic knee pain in athletes. This condition may present as a limitation in knee range of motion (ROM) due to pain or mechanical blocking [1−4]. A ganglion cyst contains a mucin-rich fluid surrounded by a pseudomembrane.

These cysts are difficult to diagnose clinically as they are not palpable. The incidence of intraarticular ganglia cyst of the knee has been reported to range from 0.20% to 1.33% on knee magnetic resonance imaging (MRI) and 0.6%−2% on knee arthroscopy [5,6]. Almost 62% of them are located on the ACL. Other frequent locations are knee collateral ligaments and posterior cruciate ligament. ACL ganglion cyst coexists with ACL mucoid degeneration in about 35% of cases (Fig. 8.1).

The mean age of patients with ACL ganglion has been reported to be 39 years old [7], although isolated cases in children aged between 2 and 12 years old have been reported in the literature [8,9]. Male preponderance has been reported and no genetic predisposition has been described [10].

The exact pathogenesis of ACL ganglion cyst is still controversial. Theories proposing to explain this condition include mucinous degeneration of connective tissue mediated by the local release of hyaluronic acid, displacement of synovial tissue during embryogenesis, and herniation of synovium into a defect of the surrounding tissue [10,11]. There are no fixed groups of symptoms that are pathognomonic of this condition and it is often discovered incidentally on MRI or knee arthroscopy while investigating painful and stiff knees.

MRI remains the gold standard imaging technique for evaluating an ACL ganglion cyst [12,13].

The treatment is essentially arthroscopic with excellent results [14].

1.2 Clinical Study

1.2.1 Symptoms

There are no specific groups of symptoms that are used to diagnose ACL ganglion cyst. These lesions should be suspected in patients with chronic knee pain and limitations in knee ROM.

Isolated ACL ganglion that is alone responsible for knee symptoms without any concomitant intraarticular pathology is regarded as "symptomatic," while incidentally detected ACL ganglion cysts associated with other knee lesions are classified as "asymptomatic" and are not necessarily responsible for the painful symptoms.

The most common presentation is chronic knee pain of insidious onset. This pain is worsened by extreme knee movements. Duration of symptoms can range from weeks-to-months and sometimes years [15]. Mechanical locking, clicking sensation, and stiffness also occur frequently. A ganglion cyst that is located anteriorly to the tibial attachment results in extension limitation, while a cyst that is located posteriorly produces flexion limitation [16,17]. There is commonly no history of knee instability.

These symptoms are mostly of spontaneous onset without a history of trauma. When trauma is reported, it is usually minor and of little significance.

1.2.2 Physical examination

The clinical examination may reveal knee joint effusion [18].

Joint line tenderness can be present on palpation of the medial and lateral aspects of the knee [19,20].

Limping and decreased gait speed can be observed and are related to pain intensity [18].

Active and passive knee ROM can have a certain limitation [19,20].

The ACL stability tests such as the anterior drawer test (Fig. 8.2), Lachman test (Fig. 8.3), and pivot shift Tests (Fig. 8.4) are negative.

Knee Pain in Sports Medicine. https://doi.org/10.1016/B978-0-323-88069-5.00001-9

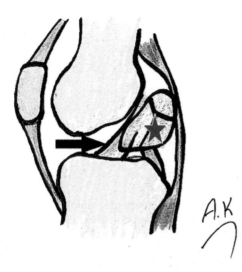

FIG. 8.1 Drawing illustrating an ACL ganglion cyst. This sagittal view demonstrates a multiloculated cyst (star) adjacent to the fibers of the ACL *(arrow)*.

1.3 Differential Diagnosis

1.3.1 Popliteal cysts

The patient usually presents with posterior knee pain and a limitation in knee ROM can be found on physical examination.

1.3.2 Knee bursitis

The patient will usually complain of local pain, tenderness, or swelling in the site of the affected bursae.

1.4 Imaging

1.4.1 Conventional X-rays

There are no specific signs of ACL ganglion cyst on conventional X-rays.

1.4.2 CT scan and arthrography

Both of these radiological examinations are specific, but they are of low diagnostic value because of their lack of sensitivity.

1.4.3 Magnetic resonance imaging

MRI scan is the gold standard investigation because of its multiplanar capability, superior identification, and morphologic interpretation of synovial tissue and ability to detect other intraarticular pathologies. It is sensitive, specific, noninvasive, and useful in planning operative treatment.

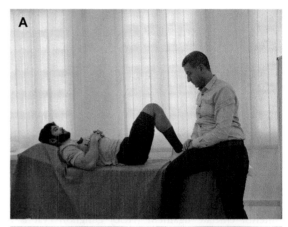

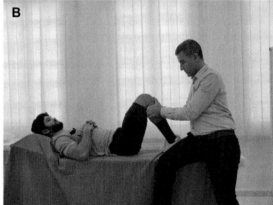

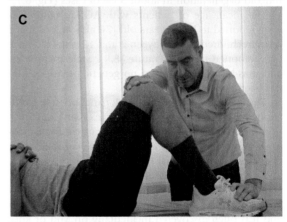

FIG. 8.2 **Pictures Illustrating the Anterior Drawer Test.** Starting position with the patient lying supine with his knee flexed (A), the examiner exerts pulling forces on the proximal end of the tibia while stabilizing the ankle (B), finally, with the knees flexed, the examiner verifies the alignment between both anterior tibial tuberosities (C).

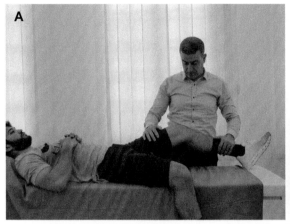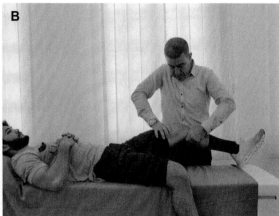

FIG. 8.3 **Pictures Illustrating the Lachman Test.** Starting position with the patient lying supine while the examiner performs slight flexion of the knee (A), the examiner exerts anteroposterior translation forces on the knee (B).

An ACL ganglion cyst appears as a fusiform or rounded structure. This structure is surrounded by a clear boundary extending along the course of the ligament. ACL ganglion cyst shows as hypointense signals on T1-weighted images and as hyperintense signals on T2-weighted images (Fig. 8.5).

Bergin defined MRI diagnostic criteria for ACL ganglion cyst [21]. Fluid signal in the substance of the ligament with at least two of the three following criteria have to be present in order to be able to retain the diagnosis.

1 Mass effect on normal ACL fibers
2 Ligament signal stronger than joint fluid
3 Lobulated aspect with definite margins

Associated internal lesions such as meniscal tear and articular cartilage damage have been reported in 22% −50% of patients [22].

1.5 Treatment
1.5.1 Conservative management
1.5.1.1 Medical treatment. Pain killers and nonsteroidal antiinflammatory drugs (NSAIDs) may be indicated by clinicians and can play a role in reducing the perceived pain. Pain response to these treatments is only partial.

1.5.1.2 Rehabilitation. A well-conducted rehabilitation program should be undertaken by the patients before and after surgery.

Such program should focus on pain management and gain in ROM while maintaining the flexibility of lower limb muscles.

Strengthening programs for the lower extremities play a role in pain management before surgery and are essential after surgical management in order to facilitate recovery.

1.5.2 Procedures
Computed tomography (CT) scan and an ultrasound (US)-guided aspiration have been tried with excellent results [23]. This procedure is reported to provide instant relief of pain and improvement in ROM. However, there are concerns about the possibility of recurrence since it is impossible to completely remove the sac of the cyst. To the best of our knowledge, no recurrence has been reported after percutaneous treatment. Another drawback of this method is the inability to address associated intraarticular pathologies. This method may only be considered in select cases of symptomatic ACL ganglion cysts. Campagnolo [23] reported the use of CT scan aspiration in athletes. An 18-gauge needle was used and local anesthetic was given to the patients. A resolution of the pain and the locking sensation of the knee was observed almost immediately.

1.5.3 Surgical treatment
Arthroscopic decompression with debridement of the cyst is the treatment of choice for instant relief of pain, improvement in ROM, and return to play.

At arthroscopy, ACL ganglion cyst appears as a cystic mass with defined margin on the ligament.

Arthroscopy allows complete excision of the cyst, along with diagnosis and treatment of other associated

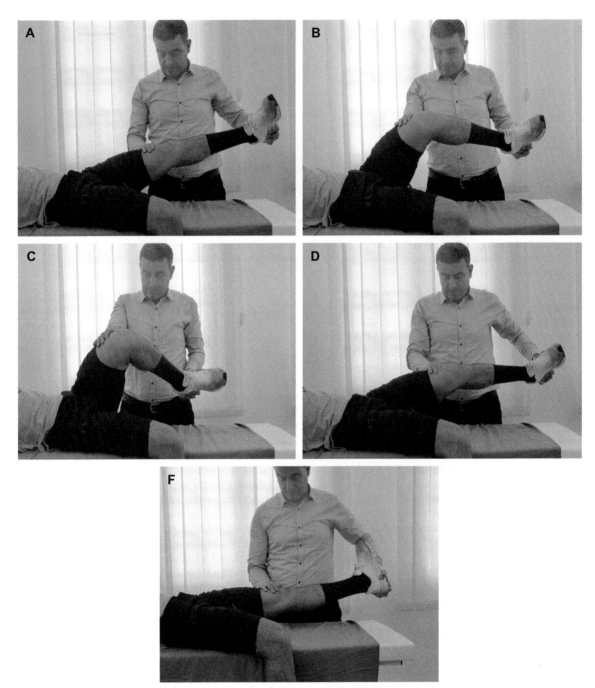

FIG. 8.4 Pictures illustrating the pivot shift test.

intraarticular knee disorders. No recurrence of symptoms or cyst on MRI postarthroscopic excision has been reported in the literature with five years as the longest follow-up [24,25].

2 ACL MUCOID DEGENERATION

2.1 Background

ACL mucoid degeneration is an uncommon knee overuse injury in athletes. The pathogenesis, the prevalence,

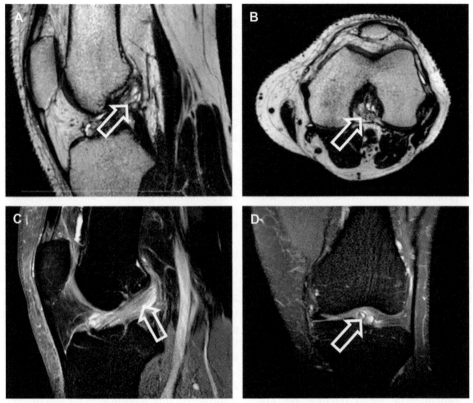

FIG. 8.5 MRI sequences of the knee in T2 sagittal and axial sections (A, B) and proton density FAT SAT sagittal (C) and coronal (D) sections illustrating a hyperintense signal (*arrows*) in relation to an ACL ganglion cyst.

and the association with other intraarticular knee structural damage are still poorly estimated.

This condition often presents with progressive knee pain, restriction in ROM without a significant history of trauma, and without knee instability.

It is characterized by degeneration of collagen fibers of the ligament and deposition of new glycosaminoglycans [25].

With the use of MRI to evaluate the painful knee joint conditions, ACL mucoid degeneration is increasingly being diagnosed incidentally. The prevalence of this condition on MRI of the knee is about 4.3% and the median age of diagnosis is 43 years old [26].

The pathogenesis of ACL mucoid degeneration is still unclear, but previous knee injury, ganglion cyst, and the degenerative process leading to the loss of synovial lining of the ACL have been suggested [27].

It was also reported that ACL mucoid degeneration might be due to repeated microtrauma. However, in

older patients, it could be due to progressive degenerative ACL lesion with a concomitant meniscal lesion.

Treatment is mainly surgical.

2.2 Clinical Study

2.2.1 Symptoms

Insidious onset of chronic knee pain located behind the patella is the most common complaint [28,29].

Symptoms can last weeks to months.

Pain may limit the movements of the knee in maximal degrees of flexion or extension. There is usually no history of significant trauma, and when present, it is normally minor. Pain and limitation in ROM have been attributed to both increased volume and tension within the ligament [30].

Locking and grinding sensations may be present.

2.2.2 Physical examination

Clinical examination may show limitation of ROM, joint line tenderness, and joint swelling. A positive grinding test of the meniscus may be present in case of concomitant meniscus injury [31].

The Lachman test, anterior drawer test, and pivot shift test for ACL integrity are usually negative.

These clinical features, however, are not pathognomonic for ACL mucoid degeneration as they are common presentations of internal knee derangement. However, they should raise suspicion and prompt further evaluation with MRI especially if the symptoms are nonspecific and resistant to NSAIDs and physiotherapy.

2.3 Differential Diagnosis

ACL mucoid degeneration can be mistakenly diagnosed as ACL rupture on MRI.

2.4 Imaging

2.4.1 Standard X-rays

Conventional X-rays will reveal potentially associated osteoarthritic changes, but they do not have any specific role in the diagnosis of ACL mucoid degeneration.

2.4.2 Magnetic resonance imaging

MRI is the main radiological investigation in the diagnosis of ACL mucoid degeneration. The MRI features of ACL mucoid degeneration are abnormal thickening of the ACL, an increased intraligamentous signal on all sequences (intermediate signal intensity on T1-weighted images, high signal intensity on T2-weighted images, and proton density weighted images) and maintenance of normal orientation and continuity of the ligament (Fig. 8.6).

ACL mucoid degeneration coexists with ACL ganglion cyst, and there is a higher association of ACL mucoid degeneration with a meniscal tear, chondral damage, and intraosseous cysts at the femoral and tibial attachment of the ligament.

2.5 Treatment

2.5.1 Conservative management

2.5.1.1 Medical treatment. Pain and limitation in ROM of the knee due to mucoid degeneration do not respond well to NSAIDs and analgesics [32].

2.5.1.2 Rehabilitation. Rehabilitation based on ROM and strengthening exercises may be attempted in association with physical modalities such as cryotherapy to reduce pain.

The current data do not support their use since it has been reported that symptoms do not respond well to physical therapy.

2.5.2 Procedures

Unlike ACL ganglion cyst, where CT scan and US-guided cyst aspiration is an effective treatment option, the interstitial nature of mucoid degeneration prevents this method from being used.

2.5.3 Surgical treatment

Arthroscopic intervention with the aim of removing the lesion without compromising the integrity of the ACL is the treatment of choice.

On arthroscopy, the ACL mucoid cyst is viewed as homogenous and hypertrophied with increased

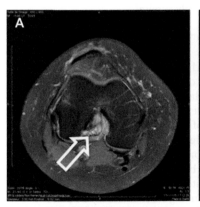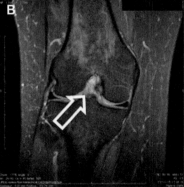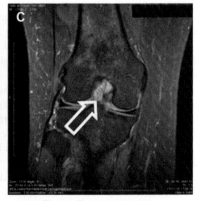

FIG. 8.6 MRI of the right knee without Cadolinium injection, in axial (A) and coronal (B and C) proton density FAT SAT sections showing global thickening of the ACL in hyper intense DP FAT SAT signal without rupture. The limits and orientation of the ligament are normal in relation to ACL mucoid degeneration. Note the absence of intraarticular effusion or osteochondral lesion.

diameter, fibers are intact with normal orientation, the synovial lining shining is lost, and a yellow mucoid substance flows upon probing [10].

The arthroscopic treatment consists of debridement and partial resection of the suffering portion of the ACL, leaving intact the rest of the anteromedial and posterolateral border and intact tibial and femoral attachments [33].

Partial resection of the ACL results in immediate relief of pain and improvement in ROM. The patient can immediately start full-weight-bearing and return to activity very soon. Aggressive total resection of the entire lesion is not supported in the literature because it has been associated with a longer delay in recovery [10]. To the best of our knowledge, there has been no recorded case of recurrence after partial resection in the literature.

2.6 Take Home Messages

Ganglion cyst and mucoid degeneration of the ACL are encountered in athletes and nonathletes.

The clinical presentation is characterized by chronic knee pain and terminal ROM limitation.

US and MRI allow diagnosis considering the lack of clinical presentation specificity.

Unlike the majority of overuse knee pain etiologies, a conservative management of these two entities is not sufficient.

The arthroscopic resection allows an immediate resolution of symptoms resulting in a prompt functional recovery without compromising the integrity of the ligament.

REFERENCES

[1] Fealy S, Kenter K, Dines JS, Warren RF. Mucoid degeneration of the anterior cruciate ligament. Arthrosc J Arthrosc Relat Surg 2001;17(9):1—4.

[2] Makino A, Pascual-Garrido C, Rolón A, Isola M, Muscolo DL. Mucoid degeneration of the anterior cruciate ligament: MRI, clinical, intraoperative, and histological findings. Knee Surg Sports Traumatol Arthrosc 2011; 19(3):408—11.

[3] Parish EN, Dixon P, Cross MJ. Ganglion cysts of the anterior cruciate ligament: a series of 15 cases. Arthrosc J Arthrosc Relat Surg 2005;21(4):445—7.

[4] Garcia-Alvarez F, Garcia-Pequerul JM, Avila JL, Sainz JM, Castiella T. Ganglion cysts associated with cruciate ligaments of the knee: a possible cause of recurrent knee pain. Acta Orthop Belg 2000;66(5):490—4.

[5] Bui-Mansfield LT, Youngberg RA. Intraarticular ganglia of the knee: prevalence, presentation, etiology, and management. AJR Am J Roentgenol 1997;168(1): 123—7.

[6] Willis-Owen CA, Konyves A, Martin DK. Bilateral ganglion cysts of the cruciate ligaments: a case report. J Orthop Surg 2010;18(2):251—3.

[7] Sayampanathan AA, Koh THB, Lee KT. Anterior cruciate ligament ganglion causing flexion restriction: a case report and review of literature. Ann Transl Med 2016; 4(11).

[8] Kakutani K, Yoshiya S, Matsui N, Yamamoto T, Kurosaka M. An intraligamentous ganglion cyst of the anterior cruciate ligament after a traumatic event. Arthrosc J Arthrosc Relat Surg 2003;19(9):1019—22.

[9] Mao Y, Dong Q, Wang Y. Ganglion cysts of the cruciate ligaments: a series of 31 cases and review of the literature. BMC Muscoskel Disord 2012;13(1):137.

[10] Lintz F, Pujol N, Boisrenoult P, Bargoin K, Beaufils P, Dejour D. Anterior cruciate ligament mucoid degeneration: a review of the literature and management guidelines. Knee Surg Sports Traumatol Arthrosc 2011; 19(8):1326—33.

[11] Krudwig WK, Schulte KK, Heinemann C. Intra-articular ganglion cysts of the knee joint: a report of 85 cases and review of the literature. Knee Surg Sports Traumatol Arthrosc 2004;12(2):123—9.

[12] Matrawy KA, El-Nekeidy AEAM, Al-Dawody A. Mucoid degeneration of the anterior cruciate ligament: frequently under-diagnosed entity in MRI. Egypt J Radiol Nucl Med 2012;43(2):227—33.

[13] Plotkin BE, Agarwal VK, Varma R. Anterior cruciate ligament ganglion cyst. Radiol Case Rep 2009;4(3).

[14] Pedrinelli A, Castellana FB, Fontes RB de V, Coelho RF. Anterior cruciate ligament ganglion: case report. Sao Paulo Med J 2002;120(6):195—7.

[15] Lunhao B, Yu S, Jiashi W. Diagnosis and treatment of ganglion cysts of the cruciate ligaments. Arch Orthop Trauma Surg 2011;131(8):1053—7.

[16] Sloane J, Gulati V, Penna S, Pastides P, Baghla DPS. Large intra-articular anterior cruciate ligament ganglion cyst, presenting with inability to flex the knee. Case Rep Med 2010;2010.

[17] Rolf C, Watson TP. Case report: intra-tendinous ganglion of the anterior cruciate ligament in a young footballer. J Orthop Surg 2006;1(1):11.

[18] Krishnamurthy A, Soraganvi P, Kumar J, Naik P. Ganglion cyst of knee associated with anterior cruciate ligament: a report of three cases. Saudi J Sports Med 2014;14(2). 99—99.

[19] Mittal S, Singla A, Nag HL, Meena S, Lohiya R, Agarwal A. Dual ACL ganglion cysts: significance of detailed arthroscopy. Case Rep Orthop 2014;2014.

[20] Sumen Y, Ochi M, Deie M, Adachi N, Ikuta Y. Ganglion cysts of the cruciate ligaments detected by MRI. Int Orthop 1999;23(1):58—60.

[21] Bergin D, Morrison WB, Carrino JA, Nallamshetty SN, Bartolozzi AR. Anterior cruciate ligament ganglia and mucoid degeneration: coexistence and clinical correlation. Am J Roentgenol 2004;182(5):1283—7.

[22] Ryan RS, Munk PL. Radiology for the surgeon: musculoskeletal case 31. Can J Surg 2004;47(1):54.

[23] Campagnolo DI, Davis BA, Blacksin MF. Computed tomography—guided aspiration of a ganglion cyst of the anterior cruciate ligament: a case report. Arch Phys Med Rehabil 1996;77(7):732—3.

[24] Sonnery-Cottet B, Guimarães TM, Daggett M, Pic JB, Kajetanek C, de Padua VBC, et al. Anterior cruciate ligament ganglion cyst treated under computed tomography—guided aspiration in a professional soccer player. Orthop J Sports Med 2016;4(5): 2325967116644585.

[25] Kwee RM, Ahlawat S, Kompel AJ, Morelli JN, Fayad LM, Zikria BA, et al. Association of mucoid degeneration of anterior cruciate ligament with knee meniscal and cartilage damage. Osteoarthr Cart 2015;23(9): 1543—50.

[26] Rossi FSF, Limbucci N, Pistoia M, Barile A, Masciocchi C. Mucoid metaplastic-degeneration of anterior cruciate ligament. J Sports Med Phys Fit 2008;48:483—7.

[27] Chudasama CH, Chudasama VC, Prabhakar MM. Arthroscopic management of mucoid degeneration of anterior cruciate ligament. Indian J Orthop 2012;46(5):561.

[28] Narvekar A, Gajjar S. Mucoid degeneration of the anterior cruciate ligament. Arthrosc J Arthrosc Relat Surg 2004; 20(2):141—6.

[29] Kumar A, Bickerstaff DR, Grimwood JS, Suvarna SK. Mucoid cystic degeneration of the cruciate ligament. J Bone Joint Surg Br March 1, 1999;81-B(2):304—5.

[30] Kim TH, Lee DH, Lee SH, Kim JM, Kim CW, Bin SI. Arthroscopic treatment of mucoid hypertrophy of the anterior cruciate ligament. Arthrosc J Arthrosc Relat Surg June 1, 2008;24(6):642—9.

[31] Pandey V, Suman C, Sharma S, Rao SP, Kiran Acharya K, Sambaji C. Mucoid degeneration of the anterior cruciate ligament: management and outcome. Indian J Orthop 2014;48(2):197—202.

[32] Hensen JJ, Coerkamp EG, Bloem JL, Schepper AMD. Mucoid degeneration of the anterior cruciate ligament. 3.

[33] Khanna G, Sharma R, Bhardwaj A, Gurdutta HS, Agrawal DK, Rathore AS. Mucoid degeneration of the anterior cruciate ligament: partial arthroscopic debridement and outcomes. J Arthrosc Jt Surg January 1, 2016; 3(1):28—33.

CHAPTER 9

Osteochondritis Dissecans

1 BACKGROUND

Osteochondritis dissecans (OCD) of the knee is a focal abnormality that affects the subchondral bone. It can cause knee instability by a detachment of bone and cartilage fragments resulting in a progression to osteoarthritis.

The incidence of this condition is estimated at 9.5/100,000 [1]. The diagnosis may be made in adult athletes and children between the ages of 12 and 19 years [2]. Epidemiological data indicate a mean age at diagnosis of 16.5 years [1]. OCD has never been diagnosed in children younger than 6 years old. The risk of developing this nontraumatic knee condition is 3.8 times higher in boys than in girls [1].

It has been reported that the terms "open physes" and "closed physes" should be preferred over the terms "juvenile" and "adult" osteochondritis [1]. Despite advances in understanding this condition, many questions remain unanswered, particularly regarding the pathophysiology, indications for magnetic resonance imaging (MRI), signs of instability, and treatment methods.

Both recreational and professional athletes may be affected by OCD. The most common site for this injury is the medial femoral condyle. The lateral femoral condyle and patella are affected less often and the tibial plateau is very rarely involved [3].

Microtraumatic origin is by far the most supported pathophysiologic mechanism [4−6].

Several risk factors were reported in the literature. In young baseball players, who frequently perform a squatted position, a study showed that the OCD lesions were located more posteriorly on the femoral condyle [7]. Some authors pointed out the close relationships between the development of OCD and the femoral posterior cruciate ligament insertion [8,9]. A study has reported that a distal location of the insertion of the posterior cruciate ligament may amplify repetitive traction stress and result in the development of OCD [10].

This microtrauma-induced mechanism may result in uneven growth in young athletes with the production of irregular subchondral bone. Patients with lateral condyle OCD often have a discoid meniscus responsible for repetitive abnormal stress [11].

OCD can heal spontaneously or worsen over time. In patients with open physes, younger age is associated with a higher chance of healing with conservative management [9].

If the lesion fails to heal, the patient experiences intermittent pain which may last for years until the fragment becomes unstable. This event is a turning point in the course of OCD, after which osteoarthritis will develop inevitably.

Younger athletes should be monitored until the radiographs are completely normal, since progression of the lesion may resume after years of latency.

Age is a key prognostic factor and OCD lesions diagnosed in adulthood are latent lesions [1]. Outcomes are better in patients with open physes [3]. Another major determinant is the surface area of the lesion since better outcomes were seen in patients with smaller surface lesions [12]. MRI visibility of a lesion measuring 1.3 mm or more in diameter predicts poor outcome [13].

2 SYNONYMS

Chondromalacia of the patella.

Articular cartilage disorder.

Unspecified internal knee derangement.

Chondromalacia of medial or lateral compartments of the knee.

Knee chondral injuries.

3 CLINICAL STUDY

3.1 Symptoms

Patients with OCD typically present with pain and swelling of variable amounts.

Pain is generally vague, poorly localized in the knee region, and exacerbated by exercise and stair climbing. Patients may present with an antalgic gait, especially in external rotation, and may report a history of multiple knee effusions [4].

Maximal tenderness is elicited over the anteromedial aspect of the knee during flexion motion. This corresponds to the most common site of OCD lesions on the lateral aspect of the distal medial femoral condyle [6].

Knee Pain in Sports Medicine. https://doi.org/10.1016/B978-0-323-88069-5.00005-6

As the lesion progresses, mechanical symptoms such as catching, locking, and giving way appear and increase in frequency and intensity, usually indicating the presence of an unstable fragment [8].

The presence of an atrophy of the quadriceps muscles of the athlete usually indicates the chronicity of symptoms [14] (Fig. 9.1).

The functional impact of OCD is usually moderate compared to other overuse knee injuries [15].

3.2 Physical Examination

A thorough physical examination must be performed as the pain may be related to a concomitant injury.

Femorotibial alignment in the sagittal plane should be assessed as medial condyle OCD is associated with varus and lateral condyle OCD with valgus of the knee [16].

Palpation of the femoral condyle at various degrees of knee flexion may trigger the patient's usual pain.

3.2.1 The Wilson test

This test consists in bending the knee at 90° then passively moving it to 30° of flexion while rotating the foot medially [9].

If the usual pain occurs during the test and resolves when the foot is rotated laterally, the test is positive. The Wilson test detects only medial condyle lesions and has only a positive predictive value. This test is a helpful diagnostic and follow-up tool.

A joint effusion [3] or a sudden increase in pain intensity while performing this test suggests an unstable lesion.

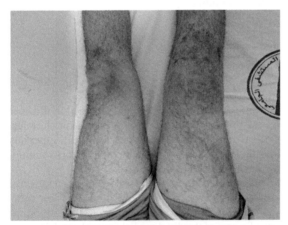

FIG. 9.1 Photograph of lower limbs showing a size difference between thighs, the right quadriceps of the patient is atrophied.

4 DIFFERENTIAL DIAGNOSIS

4.1 Meniscal Tear

A history of knee trauma is frequently found and meniscal tests are positive.

4.2 ACL Tear

The patient reports a feeling of instability and ligamentous tests are commonly positive on examination.

4.3 Osteoarthritis

Knee swelling, tenderness of the joint line, and limitation of knee ROM are suggestive of osteoarthritis. Standard knee radiographs allow diagnosis confirmation.

4.4 Plica Syndrome

The main symptom of plica syndrome is knee pain localized at the anterior aspect of the knee that is worsened when using the stairs, squatting, or bending and a catching or locking sensation can be felt when extending the knee.

5 IMAGING

5.1 Standard X-rays

Conventional radiography is the first step of the imaging study. An anteroposterior view, a lateral view, and a view with the knee flexed at 60° should be obtained. A sunrise view is required if an OCD lesion of the patella or femoral trochlea is suspected [2]. As OCD is bilateral in about 15% of cases, radiographs of the asymptomatic knee should be taken (Fig. 9.2).

A classification for OCD based on radiographic findings was described in 1988 [17] and modified in 2005 to increase accuracy [1]. The stages are focal lucency, attached fragment, and detached fragment. The stage is defined based on the bone trabecula abnormalities, without taking into consideration the condition of the overlying cartilage and viability of the fragment (Fig. 9.3).

5.2 Magnetic Resonance Imaging

MRI is the gold standard imaging modality in OCD, but it is not performed routinely. This imaging technique is indicated as a first-line examination in boys older than13 years and girls older than 11 years as well as in all patients with persistent pain despite nonoperative treatment.

It confirms the radiographic diagnosis by visualizing the fragment, which is usually hypointense on T1 images and heterogeneous on T2 images [17].

MRI may show an osteochondral fragment extending beyond the normal epiphyseal contour, a defect at

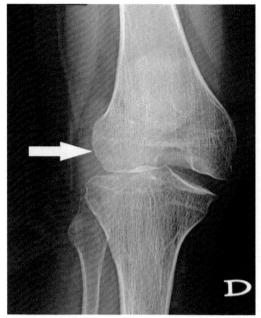

FIG. 9.2 Anteroposterior radiograph of the right knee showing a well-defined lucent image of the lateral femoral condyle (*arrow*).

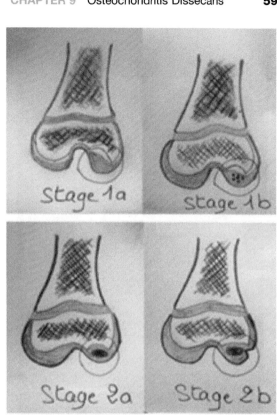

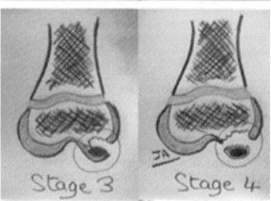

the site facing the fragment, or loose fragments within the joint cavity. Other findings include a jigsaw-puzzle appearance of the subchondral bone and spicules of the surface cartilage [17] (Figs. 9.4 and 9.5).

The surface cartilage must be examined in detail since an abnormal surface cartilage is considered as a factor of poor outcome after treatment [19]. At an advanced stage of the disease, cracks may develop into the cartilage, generating flaps or defects.

Instability is the key factor to determine the prognosis and treatment decisions. It can be evaluated based on four criteria on T2 images [20]:
- high-signal intensity line beneath the lesion
- cystic area beneath the lesion
- high-signal intensity line through the articular cartilage
- focal articular defect.

6 TREATMENT

6.1 Conservative Management

When the diagnosis is incidental, no treatment is needed but follow-up should be provided until radiographic healing is obtained.

FIG. 9.3 Radiographic classification developed by Bedouelle. Stage Ia: Defect seen as a well-defined lucent image whose contours are thickened and slightly opaquer. Stage Ib: Defect containing calcifications, which are often multiple. Stage IIa: Nodule seen as a denser and sometimes irregular image separated from the bed by a lucent line. Stage IIb: Nodule with an intraoperatively visible, thin, short fissure. Stage III or sleigh-bell aspect: Sequestered lesion that is denser, sometimes lamellar, and often demarcated from the surface of the condyle. The sequester remains anchored to the bed. Stage IV: Loose body that is completely free within the joint cavity [18].

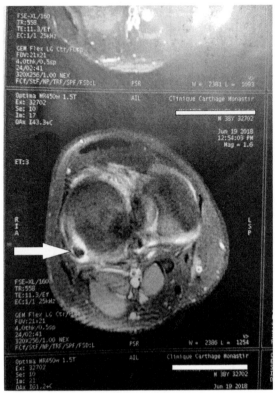

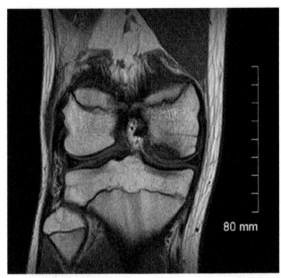

FIG. 9.5 Magnetic resonance imaging, coronal view, T1-weighted sequence: low-signal fragment within the subchondral bone.

FIG. 9.4 Magnetic resonance imaging, axial view, proton density sequence with fat-signal suppression: fragment protruding beyond the epiphyseal contour with disappearance of the overlying surface cartilage.

In patients with open physes who experience pain but have no evidence of instability, nonoperative treatment for 3−6 months should be the first option.

6.1.1 Activity modification
The importance of restricting sports activities is universally recognized. Pivoting, jumping, and repeated impacts should be avoided as well as any activity that causes the pain.

Depending on the location of the lesion, stopping specific activities for 6−8 weeks may be sufficient. If the patient fails to reduce activity, immobilization with a leg cast is useful [2].

A gradual return to sports with supervised beginning of running and jumping is allowed in the absence of knee symptoms.

It has been reported that restricting sports activities was nearly always sufficient to ensure clinical and radiographic healing after a mean follow-up of 8 months [9].

6.1.2 Medical treatment
Antiinflammatories such as nonsteroidal antiinflammatory drugs (NSAIDs) and analgesics such as paracetamol are usually helpful for short-term pain relief.

6.1.3 Rehabilitation
Early physical therapy is recommended to improve joint range of motion (ROM) and muscle strength. The focus should lie on quadriceps and hamstrings strengthening and stretching exercises. Most cartilage injuries are associated with other injuries and therefore the rehabilitation protocol should be individualized based on clinical and radiological findings. Numerous studies showed an improved cartilage healing response with the use of a passive ROM and strengthening exercises [8,9]. Most physicians agree on using continuous passive motion as well as keeping the patient nonweight bearing from 6 to 12 weeks.

6.2 Procedures
If an effusion is present, aspiration will help alleviate pain and can be combined with injection of a corticosteroid and an anesthetic. Ropivacaine should be preferred over bupivacaine because animal studies reported higher toxicity levels of the latter on chondrocytes [10].

6.3 Surgical Treatment

Persistent pain after 6 months and the development of signs of instability require surgical treatment.

6.4 Arthroscopy

Arthroscopy is the main method used for the surgical treatment of OCD. The therapeutic decision is guided by the initial exploration. The International Cartilage Repair Society developed a four-grade classification based on findings from arthroscopic inspection and palpation [21]:

- Grade I: stable lesions with a continuous but softened area covered by intact cartilage.
- Grade II: lesions with partial cartilage discontinuity that are stable when probed.
- Grade III: lesions with a complete discontinuity that are not yet dislocated (dead in situ).
- Grade IV: empty defects as well as defects with a dislocated fragment or a loose fragment.

6.5 Drilling

Drilling creates new pathways in the subchondral bone through which blood vessels can penetrate the fragment. Two techniques are available, transarticular drilling and retroarticular drilling. Transarticular drilling is performed during arthroscopy [17]. The lesion is usually identified based on its gray or yellow color, isolation, and/or softer consistency when probed, compared to the adjacent white cartilage. A total of five to ten drill holes are performed.

Sports activities can be resumed after 3−6 months depending on the postoperative evolution. The only drawback of this technique is that it violates the normal surface cartilage. Good clinical outcomes were obtained in 97.5% of cases with this procedure [14].

6.6 Fragment Fixation

An unstable fragment requires fixation to ensure stability. Fixation is also indicated for loose but intact fragments with macroscopically normal surface cartilage and a layer of subchondral bone [21].

6.7 Surgical Reconstruction: Mosaic Osteochondral Transplantation

Bone and cartilage reconstruction is required when the fragment is too severely damaged to be fixed or is detached and not found. Fortunately, these situations are rare. The defect must be carefully evaluated to determine its location, surface area, and depth [1]. This information is obtained preoperatively by MRI and per-operatively using a probe. Both cartilage and bone are lost, particularly after the bed is debrided and a simple removal of the fragment will be followed by the development of osteoarthritis. The outcomes are satisfactory in the short term but deteriorate over time. A biological membrane containing a type I or type III collagen fixed by a partially autologous fibrin glue can be placed over the site of microfracture and bone grafting to enhance chondrogenesis [20].

7 TAKE HOME MESSAGES

OCD is a multifactorial condition with a predominant role for repetitive biomechanical stress load.

Patients with OCD typically present with vague knee pain. Thus a careful physical examination (including the Wilson test) is needed to make positive diagnosis.

MRI is the gold standard investigation in OCD. It is indicated in boys older than 13 years and girls older than 11 years, and when surgical treatment is considered.

A conservative management based on sports activities restriction is often sufficient to ensure healing in patients with open physes.

Surgical fixation is required when instability is found by MRI or arthroscopy. Follow-up must be provided until complete radiographic healing of the lesion.

REFERENCES

[1] Lefort G, Moyen B, Beaufils P, De Billy B, Breda R, Cadilhac C, et al. L'ostéochondrite disséquante des condyles fémoraux: analyse de 892 cas. Rev Chir Orthopédique Réparatrice Appar Mot. 2006;92(5):97−141.

[2] Kessler JI, Nikizad H, Shea KG, Jacobs Jr JC, Bebchuk JD, Weiss JM. The demographics and epidemiology of osteochondritis dissecans of the knee in children and adolescents. Am J Sports Med 2014;42(2):320−6.

[3] Hefti F, Beguiristain J, Krauspe R, Möller-Madsen B, Riccio V, Tschauner C, et al. Osteochondritis dissecans: a multicenter study of the European pediatric Orthopedic society. J Pediatr Orthop Part B 1999;8(4):231−45.

[4] Wechter JF, Sikka RS, Alwan M, Nelson BJ, Tompkins M. Proximal tibial morphology and its correlation with osteochondritis dissecans of the knee. Knee Surg Sports Traumatol Arthrosc 2015;23(12):3717−22.

[5] Chow RM, Guzman MS, Dao Q. Intercondylar notch width as a risk factor for medial femoral condyle osteochondritis dissecans in skeletally immature patients. J Pediatr Orthop 2016;36(6):640−4.

[6] Cavaignac E, Perroncel G, Thépaut M, Vial J, Accadbled F, De Gauzy JS. Relationship between tibial spine size and the occurrence of osteochondritis dissecans: an argument in favour of the impingement theory. Knee Surg Sports Traumatol Arthrosc 2017;25(8):2442−6.

[7] Mcelroy MJ, Riley PM, Tepolt FA, Nasreddine AY, Kocher MS. Catcher's knee: posterior femoral condyle

juvenile osteochondritis dissecans in children and adolescents. J Pediatr Orthop 2016;38(8).

[8] Smillie IS. Treatment of osteochondritis dissecans. J Bone Joint Surg Br May 1957;39-B(2):248–60.

[9] Cahuzac JP, Mansat C, Clément JL, Pasquie M, Gaubert J. The natural history of osteochondritis dissecans of the knee in children. Rev Chir Orthop Reparatrice Appar Mot 1988;74(Suppl. 2):121–4.

[10] Ishikawa M, Adachi N, Yoshikawa M, Nakamae A, Nakasa T, Ikuta Y, et al. Unique anatomic feature of the posterior cruciate ligament in knees associated with osteochondritis dissecans. Orthop J Sports Med 2016; 4(5):2325967116648138.

[11] Deie M, Ochi M, Sumen Y, Kawasaki K, Adachi N, Yasunaga Y, et al. Relationship between osteochondritis dissecans of the lateral femoral condyle and lateral menisci types. J Pediatr Orthop 2006;26(1):79–82.

[12] Hughston JC, Hergenroeder PT, Courtenay BG. Osteochondritis dissecans of the femoral condyles. J Bone Joint Surg Am 1984;66(9):1340–8.

[13] Krause M, Hapfelmeier A, Möller M, Amling M, Bohndorf K, Meenen NM. Healing predictors of stable juvenile osteochondritis dissecans knee lesions after 6 and 12 months of nonoperative treatment. Am J Sports Med 2013;41(10):2384–91.

[14] Tabaddor RR, Banffy MB, Andersen JS, McFeely E, Ogunwole O, Micheli LJ, et al. Fixation of juvenile osteochondritis dissecans lesions of the knee using poly 96L/4D-lactide copolymer bioabsorbable implants. J Pediatr Orthop 2010;30(1):14–20.

[15] Rothermich MA, Nepple JJ, Raup VT, O'donnell JC, Luhmann SJ. A comparative analysis of international knee documentation committee scores for common pediatric and adolescent knee injuries. J Pediatr Orthop 2016; 36(3):274–7.

[16] Jacobi M, Wahl P, Bouaicha S, Jakob RP, Gautier E. Association between mechanical axis of the leg and osteochondritis dissecans of the knee: radiographic study on 103 knees. Am J Sports Med 2010;38(7):1425–8.

[17] Bedouelle J. L'ostéochondrite disséquante des condyles fémoraux chez l'enfant et l'adolescent. Cah D'enseignement SOFCOT Expans Sci Fr. 1988:61–93.

[18] Accadbled F, Vial J, Sales de Gauzy J. Osteochondritis dissecans of the knee. Orthop Traumatol Surg Res February 1, 2018;104(1, Suppl. ment):S97–105.

[19] De Smet AA, Ilahi OA, Graf BK. Reassessment of the MR criteria for stability of osteochondritis dissecans in the knee and ankle. Skeletal Radiol 1996;25(2): 159–63.

[20] Dipaola JD, Nelson DW, Colville MR. Characterizing osteochondral lesions by magnetic resonance imaging. Arthrosc J Arthrosc Relat Surg 1991;7(1):101–4.

[21] Brittberg M, Winalski CS. Evaluation of cartilage injuries and repair. JBJS 2003;85:58–69.

CHAPTER 10

Overuse Meniscal Pathology

1 BACKGROUND

The human menisci are fibrocartilaginous structures that have bony attachments on the tibial plateau. They are connected by ligaments to each other and to the anterior cruciate ligament, the patella, and the femur. These structures are essential for joint stability, shock absorption, distribution of contact forces, and proprioception [1].

A significant number of athletes present a problem in relation to a symptomatic degenerative meniscus. With relatively poor vascular penetration, of less than one-third of the adult meniscus, healing potential in case of chronic degeneration remains low [2] (Fig. 10.1).

Meniscal tears can be classified as acute or degenerative. While acute tears are related to excessive forces applied to a normal knee and meniscus, a degenerative tear results from repetitive microtrauma on a worn-down meniscus [2]. Tears can be described according to their pattern and location. Those located in the avascular zone have a low healing potential spontaneously and after surgical repair [3]. Degenerative tears generally have a complex pattern and are predominantly found in the posterior horn and midbody of the meniscus [4].

The patient's history and physical examination are essential to determine the meniscal origin of pain, particularly with the significant incidence of simultaneous intraarticular injuries.

On physical examination, joint line tenderness, positive McMurray (Fig. 10.2) and Appley grinding tests (Fig. 10.3), and mechanical locking are highly suggestive of a meniscal injury.

Radiographs and magnetic resonance imaging (MRI) are frequently used to diagnose meniscal tears and rule out other sources of microtraumatic knee pain.

A conservative management can relieve pain and improve function of the knee. For patients with persistent symptoms after nonsurgical management, an arthroscopic treatment can provide long term pain relief.

2 SYNONYMS

Locked knee.

3 CLINICAL STUDY

3.1 Symptoms

The main symptom of degenerative meniscal pathology is a mechanical knee pain that can be accompanied by other symptoms.

Athletes suffering from this condition are typically older than 30 years and usually complain of insidious symptoms. No acute trauma is usually found [3].

Physicians should be attentive to diagnose meniscal injury in patients with knee osteoarthritis (OA) as the two conditions are frequently associated with a concomitant prevalence of 40% [5].

Typical symptoms associated with knee pain include painful clicking, popping, locking, catching, and giving way.

In some cases, meniscus tears result in decreased walking endurance and balance performance [6].

3.2 Physical Examination

Physical examination findings that are evocative of meniscus injury include joint line tenderness, positive McMurray's test, locking, and palpable or audible clicking [1].

Quadriceps atrophy may be observed a few weeks after injury.

The examiner should evaluate the contralateral knee for comparison.

Unlike acute meniscus injury, overuse meniscus pathology is rarely manifested by joint effusion.

Knee active and passive range of motion (ROM) may be limited because of a physical blocking caused by a meniscal fragment. If the injury is not displaced, active and passive ROM are usually preserved and equivalent to the contralateral knee. With knee mobilization, a clicking may be heard or felt [1].

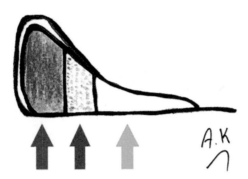

FIG. 10.1 Schematic representation of the meniscus vascularity; three zones with different vascularity can be described: red zone (*red arrow*), red white zone (*blue arrow*), and white white zone (*green arrow*).

3.3 McMurray Test

This test evaluates the medial meniscus. The patient lies supine, the knee is flexed, with the foot and tibia in external rotation. Then the foot and tibia are internally rotated and the knee is slowly extended while rotation is maintained. If pain or a click is felt, the test is considered positive.

3.4 Apley Compression Testor Meniscal Grinding Test

With the patient lying prone, the examiner flexes the knee and applies perpendicular pressure on the sole of the foot toward the examination table. The tibia is then internally and externally rotated. The test is considered positive if pain is felt.

Joint line tenderness on palpation and a positive McMurray test are described as highly suggestive of meniscus injury. Joint line tenderness sensitivity ranges from 63% to 87%, while specificity ranges from 30% to 50%. A positive McMurray test has a 32%–34% sensitivity and 78%–86% specificity [7,8].

It has been advanced that physical examination by an experienced physician has better specificity and positive predictive value than MRI for medial meniscal tears [9].

4 DIFFERENTIAL DIAGNOSIS

Differential diagnosis of degenerative meniscus injuries includes:

4.1 Anterior or Posterior Cruciate Ligament Tears

The patient reports a feeling of instability and ligamentous laxity tests are commonly present on examination.

4.2 Knee Osteoarthritis

Knee swelling, tenderness of the joint line, and limitation of knee ROM are suggestive of knee OA. Standard knee radiographs allow diagnosis confirmation.

4.3 Plica Syndromes

The main symptom of plica syndrome is knee pain localized at the anterior aspect of the knee that is worsened when using the stairs, squatting, or bending and a catching or a locking sensation felt when extending the knee.

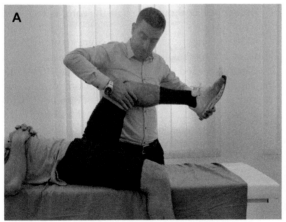
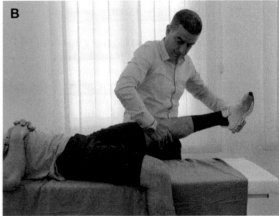

FIG. 10.2 A, B, pictures illustrating the McMurray test.

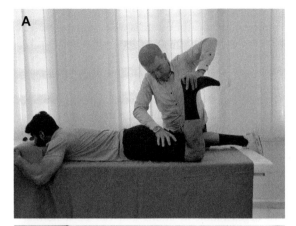

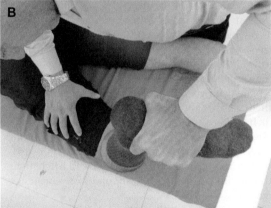

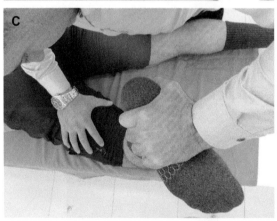

FIG. 10.3 A, B, C pictures illustrating the Appley grinding test.

4.4 Popliteal Tendinitis

Clinically, this condition is characterized by pain localized at the posterolateral aspect of the knee that appears on weight-bearing activities requiring knee flexion.

4.5 Osteochondritis Dissecans

Patients with osteochondritis dissecans (OCD) typically present with pain and swelling of variable amounts. Pain is generally vague, poorly localized in the knee region and exacerbated by exercise and stair climbing.

4.6 Fat Pad Impingement Syndrome

The patient presents with pain on either side of the patellar tendon, where the fatty tissue sits. The pain may be worse with jumping, prolonged standing, or any other position with knee hyperextension. Also, the area around the patellar tendon may be slightly swollen. Fat pad impingement is not associated with clicking, locking, or instability.

4.7 Inflammatory Arthritis

Prolonged morning stiffness, simultaneous involvement of several joints or tendons, and joint swelling may be a presentation of systemic rheumatologic joint disease.

5 IMAGING

5.1 Standard X-rays

A standard radiographic examination of the knee has a limited value in diagnosing degenerative meniscal pathology as the menisci are not visible with this technique. These radiographs are used to investigate for concomitant OA and chondrocalcinosis in older athletes [3].

5.2 Ultrasound

Ultrasound (US) examination was reported to have low value in diagnosing overuse meniscal injuries. However with the current use of dynamic US, sensitivity in detecting degenerative meniscus has reached 82% based on findings of border irregularity, cystic cavities, and calcification [10].

It has been reported that the sensitivity, specificity, and accuracy of sonography in the detection of meniscal cysts are 97%, 86%, and 94%, respectively [11].

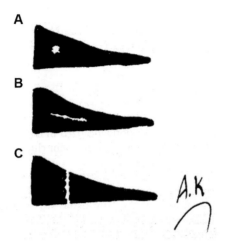

FIG. 10.4 Drawing illustrating Grades I (A) and II (B) in which an intrameniscal signal is present but does not reach the free edge. Grade III (C) has a signal change that abuts the free edge of the meniscus, indicating a meniscal tear.

On the other hand, US cannot examine deep structures of the knee with high accuracy to rule out other associated causes of knee pain.

5.3 Magnetic Resonance Imaging

MRI is the gold standard for meniscal imaging. This modality has an accuracy of 90%–95% for detecting meniscal injuries [12].

A normal meniscal structure is well evaluated on T1 sequences, while pathology is best identified on T2 sequences.

MRI signal changes related to meniscal pathology are graded from grade I to grade III [13].

Grade I signal change is intrasubstance, globular, and does not meet the articular surface.

Grade II signal change is intrasubstance, linear, and does not reach the articular surface.

Grade III changes reach the superior or inferior articular surface, or both, and represent a true tear (Figs. 10.4 and 10.5).

Grade I and II signal changes represent intrasubstance degeneration in adults and can be a normal finding related to vascular structures in children.

Recent studies have found that some grade II changes may represent a true tear [14]. MRI has the greatest sensitivity and specificity for Grade III lesions reaching 79% and 95%, respectively.

Physicians must remember to evaluate and treat the patient based on the clinical presentation along with diagnostic findings and not by imaging alone as it has been found that a 50% incidence of grade III signal changes were present in clinically asymptomatic patients over the age of 40 with OA [15]. Thus, the finding of a meniscal tear on MRI in a patient without clinical symptoms should not encourage surgery.

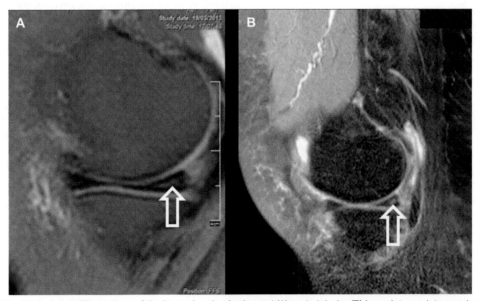

FIG. 10.5 Axial MRI sections of the knee showing horizontal (A) and globular (B) hyperintense intrameniscal signal (*arrows*) in relation to degenerative meniscal lesions.

6 TREATMENT

6.1 Conservative Management

6.1.1 Activity modification

Nonsurgical management is aimed at relieving knee pain. Patients should limit activities that trigger or exacerbate the symptoms, but complete rest is not recommended as it may result in stiffness and limitation of knee ROM.

6.1.2 Medical treatment

Nonsteroidal antiinflammatory drugs (NSAIDs) can be used on request but patients often return with incomplete symptom relief.

In the absence of contraindications, patients may need additional use for these drugs over a period of up to 6 weeks [5].

Muscle relaxants and analgesics may also be used for a short period of time in association with NSAIDs.

6.1.3 Rehabilitation

Rehabilitation is important both as conservative management and a postoperative treatment adjuvant.

A rehabilitation program should include exercises focused on maintaining ROM, improving hip and hamstring flexibility, increasing quadriceps and hip strength, and retaining knee proprioception. Recommended exercises include cycling, resisted quadriceps exercises, and squats.

Gait correction, whether by exercise or supportive orthoses, may also improve knee function and provide pain relief [16].

A well-established rehabilitation program lasting 8—12 week, followed by a home program, can provide immediate, short-term and log-term pain relief and benefits regarding mechanical symptoms up to 5 years despite the presence of degenerative joint disease progression [17].

Cryotherapy, joint mobilization, and massage can provide short-term pain relief and reduce swelling [18].

Extensor weakness remains the major problem after surgical treatment of the degenerative meniscal tear. The importance of physical therapy focused on extensor strengthening has been described [19]. Specific 3 months postoperative rehabilitation program resulted in pain relief, better knee function, and strength after a 1-year follow up [20].

6.2 Procedures

Patients presenting with an effusion may benefit from a joint aspiration to help relieve discomfort and stiffness.

In case of concomitant knee OA, injections of hyaluronic acid can be helpful [6].

6.3 Surgical Treatment

Arthroscopic partial meniscectomy can be effective in improving quality of life in patients with persistent symptoms after failure of conservative management [21].

A thorough arthroscopic evaluation of the chondral surfaces, joint spaces, and menisci is essential to determine the extent of lesions and localize meniscal tears.

Partial meniscectomy attempts to clean the unstable degenerative tear in order to create a stable tear or a smooth edge of the remaining meniscus while maintaining the meniscus as healthy as possible because complete meniscectomy may promote joint degeneration [22].

Relief from knee pain and improvement of function can be obtained quickly, 12 weeks after surgery [17]. Significant improvement in pain and knee function scores up to 5 years postoperatively has been observed [23].

Generally, the athlete may return to practice at 80% strength, typically 3—6 weeks postoperatively, and return to game competition at 90% strength, typically 5—8 weeks postoperatively [18].

7 TAKE HOME MESSAGES

Degenerative meniscus injuries are a significant source of pain for a great number of athletes.

The patient's history (including blockage and recidivant effusions), and specific clinical tests (including the McMurray test), are crucial to establish the diagnosis.

MRI allows the classification of these lesions.

Nonoperative management based on NSAID and physical therapy may provide pain relief and improve function.

In case of refractory symptoms, arthroscopic partial meniscectomy can provide short-term gains regarding pain relief, especially when followed by an effective, regular postoperative rehabilitation program.

REFERENCES

[1] Fithian DC, Kelly MA, Mow VC. Material properties and structure-function relationships in the menisci. Clin Orthop 1990;(252):19—31.

[2] Englund M, Roos EM, Roos HP, Lohmander LS. Patient-relevant outcomes fourteen years after meniscectomy: influence of type of meniscal tear and size of resection. Rheumatology 2001;40(6):631—9.

[3] Laible C, Stein DA, Kiridly DN. Meniscal repair. J Am Acad Orthop Surg April 2013;21(4):204—13.

[4] Howell R, Kumar NS, Patel N, Tom J. Degenerative meniscus: pathogenesis, diagnosis, and treatment options. World J Orthoped 2014;5(5):597.

[5] Wang CJ. Extracorporeal shockwave therapy in musculo-skeletal disorders. J Orthop Surg 2012;7(1):11.

[6] Lange AK, Singh MF, Smith RM, Foroughi N, Baker MK, Shnier R, et al. Degenerative meniscus tears and mobility impairment in women with knee osteoarthritis. Osteoarthritis Cartilage 2007;15(6):701−8.

[7] Galli M, Ciriello V, Menghi A, Aulisa AG, Rabini A, Marzetti E. Joint line tenderness and McMurray tests for the detection of meniscal lesions: what is their real diagnostic value? Arch Phys Med Rehabil June 1, 2013;94(6):1126−31.

[8] Couture JF, Al-Juhani W, Forsythe ME, Lenczner E, Marien R, Burman M. Joint line Fullness and meniscal pathology. Sport Health January 1, 2012;4(1):47−50.

[9] Ercin E, Kaya I, Sungur I, Demirbas E, Ugras AA, Cetinus EM. History, clinical findings, magnetic resonance imaging, and arthroscopic correlation in meniscal lesions. Knee Surg Sports Traumatol Arthrosc May 1, 2012;20(5):851−6.

[10] De Flaviis L, Scaglione P, Nessi R, Albisetti W. Ultrasound in degenerative cystic meniscal disease of the knee. Skeletal Radiol August 1, 1990;19(6):441−5.

[11] Rutten MJ, Collins JM, van Kampen A, Jager GJ. Meniscal cysts: detection with high-resolution sonography. Am J Roentgenol August 1, 1998;171(2):491−6.

[12] Sanders TG, Miller MD. A systematic approach to magnetic resonance imaging interpretation of sports medicine injuries of the knee. Am J Sports Med January 1, 2005;33(1):131−48.

[13] Low AK, Chia MR, Carmody DJ, Lucas P, Hale D. Clinical significance of intrasubstance meniscal lesions on MRI. J Med Imaging Radiat Oncol June 1, 2008;52(3):227−30.

[14] von Engelhardt LV, Schmitz A, Pennekamp PH, Schild HH, Wirtz DC, von Falkenhausen F. Diagnostics of degenerative meniscal tears at 3-Tesla MRI compared to arthroscopy as reference standard. Arch Orthop Trauma Surg May 1, 2008;128(5):451−6.

[15] Fukuta S, Kuge A, Korai F. Clinical significance of meniscal abnormalities on magnetic resonance imaging in an older population. Knee June 1, 2009;16(3):187−90.

[16] Elbaz A, Beer Y, Rath E, Morag G, Segal G, Debbi EM, et al. A unique foot-worn device for patients with degenerative meniscal tear. Knee Surg Sports Traumatol Arthrosc February 1, 2013;21(2):380−7.

[17] Østerås H, Østerås B, Torstensen TA. Medical exercise therapy, and not arthroscopic surgery, resulted in decreased depression and anxiety in patients with degenerative meniscus injury. J Bodyw Mov Ther October 1, 2012;16(4):456−63.

[18] Frizziero A, Ferrari R, Giannotti E, Ferroni C, Poli P, Masiero S. The meniscus tear: state of the art of rehabilitation protocols related to surgical procedures. Muscles Ligaments Tendons J January 21, 2013;2(4):295−301.

[19] Moffet H, Richards CL, Malouin F, Bravo G. Impact of knee extensor strength deficits on stair ascent performance in patients after medial meniscectomy. Scand J Rehabil Med June 1993;25(2):63−71.

[20] Østerås H, Østerås B, Torstensen TA. Is postoperative exercise therapy necessary in patients with degenerative meniscus? A randomized controlled trial with one year follow-up. Knee Surg Sports Traumatol Arthrosc January 1, 2014;22(1):200−6.

[21] Lim HC, Bae JH, Wang JH, Seok CW, Kim MK. Non-operative treatment of degenerative posterior root tear of the medial meniscus. Knee Surg Sports Traumatol Arthrosc April 1, 2010;18(4):535−9.

[22] Wilson W, van Rietbergen B, van Donkelaar CC, Huiskes R. Pathways of load-induced cartilage damage causing cartilage degeneration in the knee after meniscectomy. J Biomech June 1, 2003;36(6):845−51.

[23] Herrlin SV, Wange PO, Lapidus G, Hållander M, Werner S, Weidenhielm L. Is arthroscopic surgery beneficial in treating non-traumatic, degenerative medial meniscal tears? A five year follow-up. Knee Surg Sports Traumatol Arthrosc February 1, 2013;21(2):358−64.

CHAPTER 11

Knee Bursitis

1 BACKGROUND

Bursae are located between surfaces exposed to friction and movement, often between different types of tissues like tendons and bones. Knee bursitis is a disorder related to an inflammation of any of the bursa in the knee joint region. It is a common clinical disorder that may lead to functional impairments. The clinical presentation of a bursitis depends on its location, size, mass effect, and relationship to surrounding structures. They are often asymptomatic and may be incidentally found on inspection or imaging examinations [1]. Occasionally, they may cause pain, swelling, nerve compression, erosion, or joint impairment. In rare cases, the clinical presentation of a knee bursitis may be misleading. For example, parameniscal cysts are always associated with meniscal tears and popliteal cysts are highly associated with osteoarthritis of the medial compartment of the knee [2].

Asymptomatic knee bursitis is often treated with observation alone, while the treatment of symptomatic cysts depends on the underlying cause. Microtrauma-related bursitis is usually treated with steroid injection and immobilization. Bursitis that impairs joint function may require aspiration or resection. If a bursitis is associated with underlying joint disease, it is important to address the underlying joint abnormality to prevent recurrence [3].

Eleven bursae are found within the knee region [2] (Fig. 11.1).

Three bursae communicate with the knee joint. Four of them are associated with the patella, two are related to the semimembranosus tendons and two are related to the collateral ligaments of the knee [3].

2 CLINICAL STUDY

2.1 Symptoms

The patient usually complains of mild local pain which may be associated with swelling in the affected site. The pain is worse with flexion and usually occurs at night or after activity. In some cases, the pain may be intense and accompanied by morning stiffness [2].

Walking promptly becomes painful and limping may be present. A limitation in knee range of motion (ROM), especially in flexion, may impair driving and sitting at a desk at work.

Patients will also have problems leaning, kneeling, crawling, or climbing, which may interfere with professional and recreational activities. Athletes such as runners may have diminished performance or may be even put off play [4].

2.2 Physical Examination

The patient may have an antalgic gait, with a shortened stance phase on the affected side. There is tenderness to palpation associated with swelling at the site of the involved bursa, and there may be associated to local inflammatory signs and crepitation [3].

If the bursa connects with the knee joint, there may be an associated joint effusion.

Knee ROM is often limited by pain and increased intraarticular tension.

The neurologic examination findings should be normal.

Decreased balance is often seen in older patients, sometimes necessitating assistive devices such as a walker, crutches, cane, or even a wheelchair [4].

2.3 Topographic Forms

The most common knee bursitis conditions are the following.

2.3.1 Prepatellar bursitis (Housemaid's knee)

Prepatellar bursitis can be caused by microtrauma such as frequent kneeling on a hard surface or direct trauma, such as falling on a bent knee [3]. It has been reported to be associated with knee osteoarthritis in 3.1% of cases [4].

2.3.2 Infrapatellar bursitis (Vicar's knee)

Infrapatellar bursitis is usually due to repetitive knee flexion in weight bearing, such as deep knee bends, squatting, or jumping. It can be associated with patellar and quadriceps tendinopathies [5]. It is associated with knee osteoarthritis in 10.6% of patients [4].

Knee Pain in Sports Medicine. https://doi.org/10.1016/B978-0-323-88069-5.00006-8

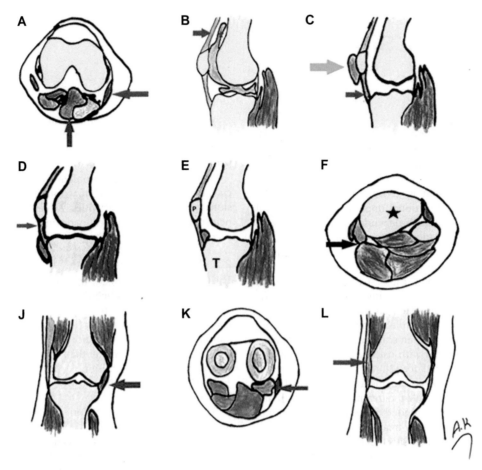

FIG. 11.1 **Drawing illustrating the most frequent bursitis of the knee:**   (A) a popliteal cyst. This axial view shows a popliteal cyst (*blue*) located between the semimembranosus tendon (*red arrow*) and the medial gastrocnemius muscle (*blue arrow*). (B) The suprapatellar bursa. This sagittal view demonstrates the suprapatellar bursa (*) located posteriorly to the quadriceps tendon (*arrowheads*) and above the patella (P). This bursa usually communicates with the knee joint. (C) Drawing illustrating a prepatellar bursitis. This sagittal view shows a fluid collection within the prepatellar bursa (*green arrow*), located anteriorly to the patella and the proximal part of the patellar tendon (*red arrow*). (D) A superficial infrapatellar bursitis. This sagittal view demonstrates a fluid collection within the superficial infrapatellar bursa (*blue*), located anteriorly to the distal part of the patellar tendon (*red arrow*), near its insertion at the tibia. (E) a deep infrapatellar bursitis. This sagittal view demonstrates a fluid collection within the deep infrapatellar bursa (*blue*), located posteriorly to the distal part of the patellar tendon, and anteriorly to the anterior aspect of the tibia (T). P—patella. (F) An anserine bursitis. This axial view shows the anserine bursa (*arrow*) located between the medial aspect of the tibia (star) and the tendons forming the pes anserinus. (J) A medial collateral ligament bursitis. This coronal view demonstrates a fluid collection (*blue arrow*) between the superficial and deep layers of this ligament. (K) A semimembranosus—medial collateral ligament bursitis. This axial view demonstrates a fluid collection in this bursa (*blue arrow*). (L) Drawing illustrating an iliotibial bursitis. This coronal view demonstrates a fluid collection within the iliotibial bursa (*red arrow*), located medially to the iliotibial band (*green*).

2.3.3 Anserine bursitis

Anserine bursitis is commonly seen in individuals who participate in sports that require running, side-to-side movement and cutting and in overweight older women with knee osteoarthritis [6]. It is responsible for 2.5% of medial knee pain [7].

2.3.4 Medial collateral ligament bursitis

Medial collateral ligament bursitis refers to inflammation of a bursa located between the deep and superficial parts of the medial collateral ligament [5]. It is associated with degenerative disease of the medial joint compartment [8]. This bursitis may be seen in horseriding and motorcycle athletes because of the friction applied to the medial side of the knee [8].

2.3.5 Semimembranosus bursitis

Semimembranosus bursitis is usually seen in runners and may be associated with hamstring tendinitis [2]. This bursitis was seen in 4.4% of subjects with knee pain explored with magnetic resonance imaging (MRI) [4].

3 DIFFERENTIAL DIAGNOSIS

Necrotic or mucinous neoplasms.

There is usually some solid component that differentiates these more serious masses from the benign cystic lesions.

4 IMAGING

The aim of knee bursitis imaging is to confirm the cystic nature of the lesion, determine its relationship with the joint and the surrounding structures, and to evaluate the joint for associated disorders.

4.1 Standard X-rays

Standard radiographs have a limited value for assessing soft tissue abnormalities. They may demonstrate soft tissue swelling, effusion, signs of associated degenerative joint disease, bone erosion, calcification, or intraarticular calcifications in case of a communicating bursa [8].

4.2 Arthrography

Arthrography can be helpful in demonstrating the communication of a cyst with the joint cavity. However, when the communication is very narrow or when the bursa is filled with highly viscous fluid, it may not be filled with the contrast product and in these cases, arthrography offers little information [6].

4.3 Ultrasound

Ultrasound (US) is adapted to study suspected bursitis. It can be used to demonstrate the location and extent of cysts and can differentiate cysts from noncystic masses. However, US has limited ability to evaluate for associated intraarticular abnormalities. Furthermore, cysts containing debris or hyperplastic synovium may simulate solid mass lesions [5] (Figs. 11.2 and 11.3).

4.4 CT Scan

Computed tomography (CT) scan is an excellent tool in assessing abnormalities of calcified tissues because of its high spatial resolution. However, its value for assessing soft tissue lesions is limited by its low soft tissue contrast. Paraarticular cysts are of lower attenuation than muscle and of higher attenuation than fat, and lack of enhancement will be seen following intravenous contrast administration [7].

4.5 Magnetic Resonance Imaging

MRI is superior to all other imaging modalities for investigating soft tissue abnormalities, particularly for demonstrating the location and extent of the lesion. MRI offers superior soft tissue contrast and multiplanar imaging capabilities and is noninvasive [5]. MRI may show the exact location of the bursitis and study its relationship to the joint and surrounding structures. The lack of enhancement after injection confirms the cystic nature of the lesion. In addition, MRI imaging is very accurate in detecting associated joint disorders, such as meniscal tears, ligamentous abnormalities, and degenerative or inflammatory changes [5] (Fig. 11.4).

5 TREATMENT

5.1 Conservative Management

5.1.1 Activity modification

Initial restriction of activity that provokes or aggravates symptoms is important [3,9]. In athletes, this may mean a substitution of the usual athletic activities during the healing process.

Local cryotherapy helps decrease pain and inflammation. The patient can be taught to use superficial heat for chronic bursitis. This can be done with moistened warm compresses or with a microwaveable heating pack. Precautions should be observed and given to the patient to prevent burns.

5.1.2 Medical treatment

Nonsteroidal antiinflammatory drugs (NSAIDs) can be prescribed to decrease pain and inflammation. Oral steroids are generally not indicated as initial treatment [8].

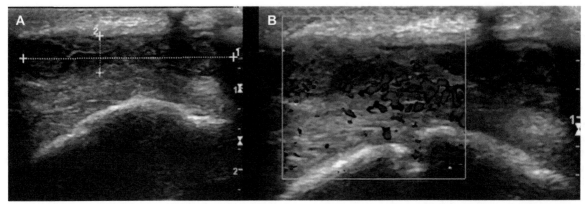

FIG. 11.2 Standard (A) and Doppler (B) knee US images illustrating a hypoechoic structure with increased Doppler signal in relation to a suprapatellar bursitis.

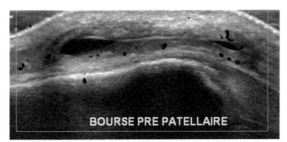

FIG. 11.3 US of the knee illustrating a hypoechoic structure with increased Doppler signal in relation to a prepatellar bursitis.

5.1.3 Rehabilitation

Physical therapy should include stretching of the quadriceps, hamstrings, iliotibial band, and hip adductor muscles if these muscles are tight [2].

Strengthening exercises are often needed in chronic knee bursitis because of disuse weakness. Correction of gait abnormalities is also important. Patients should be advised to protect their knees from further trauma by avoiding bending or kneeling and by using knee pads. Modalities such as US have not been proved to be more effective than a combination of the aforementioned measures. US should be avoided when an effusion is present because it can worsen it [10].

5.1.4 Orthoses

The use of an orthosis in the affected knee may assist in preventing painful movement and further inflammation and provide comfort. Shoe inserts unilaterally or bilaterally may have a role in the correction of altered

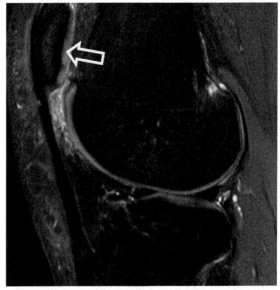

FIG. 11.4 T2-weighted sagittal MRI section of the knee showing a hyperintense signal (*arrow*) in relation to a suprapatellar bursitis.

biomechanics of the lower extremities and an improvement in symptoms.

5.2 Procedures

Aspiration is rarely needed but may be necessary if an infection is suspected.

Intrabursal corticosteroid injection is indicated if there is no response to conservative management or if the patient demonstrates significant functional limitations [6].

Typically, no more than three injections are indicated over a 6–12-month period.

The patient is generally advised to avoid activity involving the injected area for approximately 2 weeks to promote retention of the corticosteroid in the bursa and to avoid systemic absorption [11]. Some studies suggest that patients who have pes anserinus bursitis may have the best outcome after corticosteroid injection [12,13].

This injection may be guided by a high-frequency linear US transducer placed along the medial aspect of the knee, a mixture of anesthetic and long-acting corticosteroid is injected through a 25-gauge needle [14].

Chemical ablation has been used as an alternative to surgery in cases of persistent prepatellar bursitis [15].

5.3 Surgical Treatment

Surgery is generally not indicated and should be suggested only in refractory cases.

Excision of the affected bursa can be considered if the disease does not respond to conservative measures because it greatly limits the patient's activities.

Successful surgical resection of bursae has been reported in the literature [16,17]. Outpatient endoscopic bursectomy under local anesthesia has been reported as an effective treatment of prepatellar bursitis after failure of conservative management [18].

6 TAKE HOME MESSAGES

Knee bursitis is a common cause of microtraumatic knee pain in athletes.

The clinical presentation depends on the location, the size, and the relationship with surrounding tissues.

Painful knee ROM limitation associated with a joint effusion is a key symptom.

MRI is superior to US in assessing the size, the communication with the knee, and the relation to adjacent anatomical structures.

Conservative treatment should be tried in small bursitis, while surgical management is recommended in large persistent ones.

REFERENCES

[1] Le Manac'h AP, Ha C, Descatha A, Imbernon E, Roquelaure Y. Prevalence of knee bursitis in the workforce. Occup Med Oxf Engl December 2012;62(8):658–60.

[2] Larson RLR, Grana WA. The knee: Form, function, pathology, and treatment. Saunders; 1993.

[3] Cailliet R. Knee pain and disability. Internet. Philadelphia: Davis; 1988 [cited 2018 Nov 21]. Available from: https://trove.nla.gov.au/work/16350895.

[4] Hill CL, Gale DR, Chaisson CE, Skinner K, Kazis L, Gale ME, et al. Periarticular lesions detected on magnetic resonance imaging: prevalence in knees with and without symptoms. Arthritis Rheum 2003;48(10):2836–44.

[5] Biundo JJ. Regional rheumatic pain syndromes. Primer Rheum Dis 1997;12:174–87.

[6] Alvarez-Nemegyei J, Canoso JJ. Evidence-based soft tissue rheumatology IV: anserine bursitis. J Clin Rheumatol Pract Rep Rheum Musculoskelet Dis August 2004;10(4):205–6.

[7] Rennie WJ, Saifuddin A. Pes anserine bursitis: incidence in symptomatic knees and clinical presentation. Skeletal Radiol July 2005;34(7):395–8.

[8] McCarthy CL, McNally EG. The MRI appearance of cystic lesions around the knee. Skeletal Radiol April 2004;33(4):187–209.

[9] Kang I, Han SW. Anserine bursitis in patients with osteoarthritis of the knee. South Med J 2000;93(2):207–9.

[10] Johnson EW. Rehabilitation medicine principles and practice. In: Delisa JA, Currie DM, Gans BM, Gatens PF, Leonard JA, McPhee MC, et al., editors. Muscle nerve, vol. 12; May 1, 1989. p. 427–8. Philadelphia, 1988, $75.00, 1024 pp.

[11] Neustadt DH. Intra-articular corticosteroids and other agents: aspiration techniques. 1988. p. 812–25. Diagn Manag Rheum Dis Second Ed Phila PA JB Lippincott.

[12] Yoon HS, Kim SE, Suh YR, Seo YI, Kim HA. Correlation between ultrasonographic findings and the response to corticosteroid injection in pes anserinus tendinobursitis syndrome in knee osteoarthritis patients. J Kor Med Sci 2005;20(1):109–12.

[13] Handy JR. Anserine bursitis: a brief review. South Med J 1997;90(4):376–7.

[14] Jose J, Schallert E, Lesniak B. Sonographically guided therapeutic injection for primary medial (tibial) collateral bursitis. J Ultrasound Med 2011;30(2):257–61.

[15] Ike RW. Chemical ablation as an alternative to surgery for treatment of persistent prepatellar bursitis. J Rheumatol 2009;36(7). 1560–1560.

[16] Yamamoto T, Akisue T, Marui T, Hitora T, Nagira K, Mihune Y, et al. Isolated suprapatellar bursitis: computed tomographic and arthroscopic findings. Arthrosc J Arthrosc Relat Surg 2003;19(2):1–5.

[17] Klein W. Endoscopy of the deep infrapatellar bursa. Arthrosc J Arthrosc Relat Surg 1996;12(1):127–31.

[18] Huang YC, Yeh WL. Endoscopic treatment of prepatellar bursitis. Int Orthop 2011;35(3):355–8.

CHAPTER 12

Osgood–Schlatter Disease

1 BACKGROUND

Osteochondrosis of the tibial tubercle was reported for the first time in the early 1900s. Two different physicians reported pain located in the tibial tubercle that occur during sports activities involving jumping and running in active adolescents. This condition was named after Osgood and Schlatter in recognition for their work. The authors explained the syndrome by rapid growth in children and stress transmitted through patellar tendon on the developing tubercle.

The researchers declared that this condition was different from tibial tubercle avulsion fracture and reported that it is due to repetitive microtrauma [1]. Nowadays Osgood–Schlatter disease (OSD) is considered as a traction apophysitis. The primary cause of this condition is the stress from the patellar tendon at its point of insertion [2,3] (Fig. 12.1).

The retraction of the rectus femoris muscle was also reported to be one of the main factors associated with the presence of OSD in adolescents [3]. The injury mechanism in adults is usually related to direct impact on the tubercle, rather than contraction of the quadriceps as seen in adolescents [4].

Pathogenesis of this disease includes a partial loss of continuity of the patellar tendon-cartilage-bone junction at the tibial tuberosity. An inflammatory process starts in the region and results in patellar tendinitis, multiple subacute fractures, and irregular ossification.

If these patients continue sport activities, microavulsions increase over time. This may cause a separated fragment leading to a chronic pain in the front aspect of the knee [5–7].

Some studies showed that patients affected by OSD have predisposing anatomical abnormalities at the point of insertion of the patellar tendon and histological studies support the microtraumatic etiology of this condition [8,9].

OSD was originally reported to be more frequent in boys. With the increasing number of young female athletes, this syndrome is now being seen at a similar rate in both genders [4]. OSD is typically more common between the ages of 8 and 13 years in girls and between 12 and 15 years in boys [5]. It affects 21% of athletic adolescents, while it is seen in 4.5% of nonathletic controls with the same age [10,11]. The disease can be bilateral in 20%–30% of cases [4].

The individual's history and the physical examination are usually sufficient to make a diagnosis of OSD.

Treatment of this condition is mainly conservative.

2 CLINICAL STUDY

2.1 Symptoms

Patients complain of pain related to physical activities or sports. This pain is located on the tibial tubercle and distal patellar tendon. It occurs with activities and disappears with rest. It starts as a dull ache gradually increasing with activity. Pain typically improves with rest and will disappear minutes to hours after the culprit activity or sport is stopped.

It is exacerbated particularly by running, jumping, direct knee impact, kneeling, and squatting.

In general, the pain is present with activities involving stress on the knee in flexion, leading to an eccentric quadriceps contraction [5].

2.2 Physical Examination

During the acute phase of the disease, patients may walk with an antalgic gait.

On physical examination, there is usually tenderness while palpating the tibial tubercle, knee swelling, thickening of the patellar tendon, and enlargement of the tibial tuberosity (Fig. 12.2).

In chronic conditions, a firm mass or bone irregularities are often found during palpation. Acute cases may present with an active knee extension deficit.

There is no sign of effusion or instability, and passive range of motion (ROM) in the knee is usually preserved.

Quadriceps and hamstring muscle retraction is commonly found on examination [5,12].

Knee Pain in Sports Medicine. https://doi.org/10.1016/B978-0-323-88069-5.00011-1

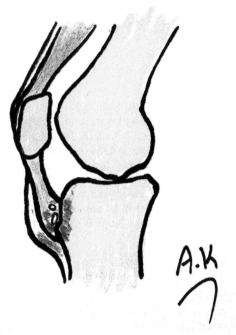

FIG. 12.1 Drawing illustrating the mechanism of OSD: As the patellar tendon exerts traction on its insertion on the tibial tubercle, inflammation and fragmentation occur.

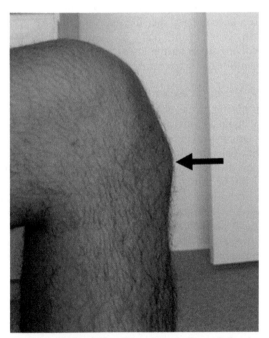

FIG. 12.2 Photograph with a lateral view of the knee showing an enlargement of the tibial tuberosity (*arrow*) in a patient with OSD sequelae.

3 DIFFERENTIAL DIAGNOSIS

The differential diagnosis of OSD includes:

3.1 Osteochondritis Dissecans

Pain is rather felt as intraarticular and patients present with a swelling of variable amounts.

3.2 Sinding Larsen Johansson Syndrome (SLJS)

Pain localized to the inferior patellar pole in a young athlete with swelling is suggestive of this condition.

3.3 Patellofemoral Pain Syndrome (PFP)

Pain is provoked by prolonged sitting and while using the stairs. On physical examination, patellar stress tests are positive.

3.4 Avulsion Fracture of the Tibial Tuberosity

A history of knee trauma is usually present.

3.5 Pes Anserinus Bursitis

Typical signs include pain in the medial aspect of the knee and edema of the site of insertion of the pes anserinus.

3.6 Tumor and Infection

Local and general inflammatory signs are suggestive of these conditions.

4 IMAGING

4.1 Standard X-rays

Standard radiographs of the knee are requested because they allow the evaluation of the tibial tuberosity.

The lateral radiograph is most helpful in evaluating the insertion of the knee's extensor system (Fig. 12.3).

A radiological evaluation may show superficial ossification in the patellar tendon, soft tissue swelling facing the anterior tibial tuberosity, and thickening of the patellar tendon.

These signs may be a normal variant in asymptomatic children, especially in the preossification phase. On the other hand, cases of incidental OSD have been diagnosed with radiography without any clinical symptoms [13].

An ossification in the patellar tendon may be rarely present with an acute knee pain and could be considered as a fracture at first [14].

A fragmentation of apophysis shows that the patient is in the chronic stage.

4.2 Ultrasound

US may show the thickened patellar tendon better than plain radiography.

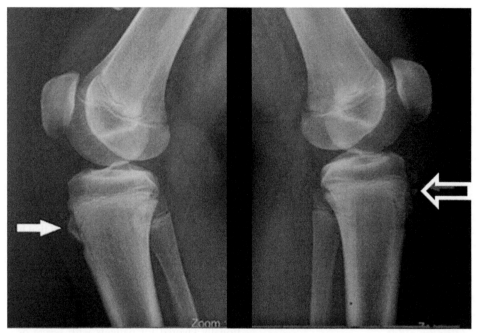

FIG. 12.3 Knee lateral radiographs showing bilateral OSD with tibial tubercle fragmentation in the right knee (*white arrow*) and intratendinous calcifications in the left knee (*empty arrow*).

It can also demonstrate pretibial swelling, fragmentation of the ossification center, and excessive fluid collection in the infrapatellar bursa [15].

4.3 Magnetic Resonance Imaging

Magnetic resonance imaging (MRI) allows for a positive diagnosis of OSD and may be more useful in revealing early and progressive lesions or atypical OSD presentations [3].

On T2-weighted imaging, a hyperintense irregular signal can be viewed (Fig. 12.4).

MRI may also play a role in evaluating the progression of the condition. An MRI study of children diagnosed with this condition classified lesions into

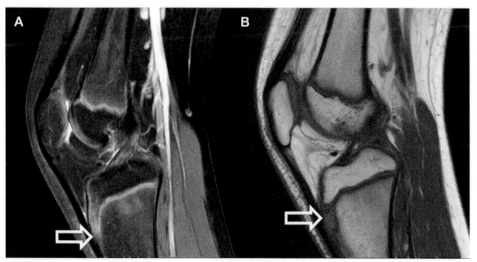

FIG. 12.4 Knee MRI in T2 (A) and T1 (B) illustrating tibial tubercule signal abnormalities (*arrows*) in relation to an OSD.

five stages. The images were classified into five stages as follows: normal, early, progressive, terminal, and healing [5].

- In the normal stage, MRI was normal, but the patient had painful symptoms.
- The early stage was defined by the presence of an inflammation around the secondary ossification center and no avulsed portion.
- The progressive stage was defined as the presence of partial cartilaginous avulsion from the secondary ossification center.
- The terminal stage was defined as the existence of separated bone fragments.
- The healing stage was defined as an ossification of the tibial tuberosity without separated fragments.

The role of MRI in diagnosis, prognosis, and management is mainly limited by accessibility to this examination [5].

5 TREATMENT

5.1 Conservative Management

5.1.1 Activity modification

The treatment of OSD is guided by the severity of the symptoms.

OSD is considered to be a self-limited disease and generally ends with skeletal maturity. Improvement will be gradual and the condition may persist for 12−18 months. Although most young athletes continue to practice sports, the severity of pain in some individuals should indicate a change in sports type or in position.

Nonimpact activities, including swimming and cycling, can be continued to maintain patient's cardiovascular fitness. Hamstrings and quadriceps flexibility exercises are useful to maintain knee ROM and may accelerate recovery.

A conservative therapy also includes knee bracing until the symptoms resolve.

A brief period of controlled immobilization may be indicated in cases of patients with high intensity pain making them unable to perform daily activities.

OSD may cause disability in the chronic stage. Patients with recurring symptoms should be regularly followed with clinical and radiological evaluations during conservative treatment [12].

Complications like pseudoarthrosis, genu recurvatum, patella alta, fragmentation/migration of the patellar tendon ossicle may occur leading to early knee osteoarthritis [16].

Despite conservative measures, 10% of patients experience persistent symptoms in adulthood [11].

5.1.2 Medical treatment

Nonsteroidal antiinflammatory drugs (NSAIDs) are generally used for a short period of time to provide pain relief and reduce local inflammation.

In particular, ibuprofen, naproxen, flurbiprofen, and ketoprofen are chosen for their analgesic, antipyretic, and antiinflammatory effects.

5.2 Procedures

In the past, some authors recommended an injection of corticosteroids into the patellar tendon to provide symptomatic relief. However, it is not recommended currently due to its deleterious effects since it can cause subcutaneous atrophy and rupture of the patellar tendon [17,18].

A study by Topol et al. [19] showed that hyperosmolar dextrose injection for a refractory OSD was helpful in reducing pain, sport modification frequency, and prompted the return to play.

5.3 Surgical Treatment

Although conservative management has been conventionally favored for patients with severe or persistent symptoms, surgical intervention can be effective [20,21].

Surgery is rarely indicated for OSD in adolescents. Research revealed that the removal of ossicle fragmentation in immature patients leads to premature fusion of the tibial tubercle [22]. Particularly, adults with continued symptoms may need surgical treatment [17].

Surgical procedures include drilling of the tubercle, removal of loose fragments, autogenous bone graft, and tibial tuberosity excision or sequestrectomy.

Surgical management of the OSD is performed through open or arthroscopic or direct bursoscopic excision [21,23,24].

The two most common procedures performed are ossicle excision and tibial tubercle prominence resection [21,25].

Ossicle removal is supposed to be the best method in the surgical treatment of OSD [23,25]. Tubercle prominence resection has also shown good results in refractory recalcitrant cases [26,27].

Procedures that promote early fusion of the apophysis of the tuberosity to the diaphysis, such as attaching the tubercle to the tibial metaphysis with autogenous bone graft or drilling the tuberosity, are not been recommended since premature fusion of the anterior part of the epiphysis leading to genu recurvatum has been reported with these interventions [28,29].

6 TAKE HOME MESSAGES

Young athletes who give a history of a rapid growth and who participate in intense sports activities are particularly affected.

The clinical presentation typically includes anterior knee pain, swelling, and tenderness involving the tibial tubercule.

Generally, OSD is a self-limiting condition. However, in some cases, symptoms may persist and painful sequelae may be observed in adult athletes.

The management is mainly conservative and surgical procedures should be reserved to refractory cases in adults.

REFERENCES

[1] Ogden JA, Southwick WO. Osgood-Schlatter's disease and tibial tuberosity development. Clin Orthop 1976; 116:180—9.

[2] Demirag B, Ozturk C, Yazici Z, Sarisozen B. The pathophysiology of Osgood—Schlatter disease: a magnetic resonance investigation. J Pediatr Orthop B 2004;13(6): 379—82.

[3] Hirano A, Fukubayashi T, Ishii T, Ochiai N. Magnetic resonance imaging of Osgood-Schlatter disease: the course of the disease. Skeletal Radiol 2002;31(6): 334—42.

[4] de Lucena GL, dos Santos Gomes C, Guerra RO. Prevalence and associated factors of Osgood-Schlatter syndrome in a population-based sample of Brazilian adolescents. Am J Sports Med 2011;39(2):415—20.

[5] Gholve PA, Scher DM, Khakharia S, Widmann RF, Green DW. Osgood Schlatter syndrome. Curr Opin Pediatr 2007;19(1):44—50.

[6] Goodier D, Maffulli N, Good J. Tibial tuberosity avulsion associated with patellar tendon avulsion. Acta Orthop Belg 1994;60. 235—235.

[7] Maffulli N, Grewal R. Avulsion of the tibial tuberosity: muscles too strong for a growth plate. Clin J Sport Med Off J Can Acad Sport Med 1997;7(2):129—32.

[8] Ehrenborg G. The Osgood-Schlatter lesion. A clinical study of 170 cases. Acta Chir Scand 1962;124:89—105.

[9] Ehrenborg G. The Osgood-Schlatter lesion: a clinical and experimental study. Acata Chir Scand Suppl 1962;288: 1—36.

[10] Dunn JF. Osgood-Schlatter disease. Am Fam Physician 1990;41(1):173—6.

[11] Kujala UM, Kvist M, Heinonen O. Osgood-Schlatter's disease in adolescent athletes: retrospective study of incidence and duration. Am J Sports Med 1985;13(4): 236—41.

[12] Çakmak S, Tekin L, Akarsu S. Long-term outcome of Osgood-Schlatter disease: not always favorable. Rheumatol Int 2014;34(1):135.

[13] Morgan B, Mullick S, Harper WM, Finlay DB. An audit of knee radiographs performed for general practitioners. Br J Radiol 1997;70(831):256—60.

[14] Yen YM. Assessment and treatment of knee pain in the child and adolescent athlete. Pediatr Clin 2014;61(6): 1155—73.

[15] Blankstein A, Cohen I, Heim M, Salai M, Chechick A, Ganel A, et al. Ultrasonography as a diagnostic modality in Osgood-Schlatter disease. Arch Orthop Trauma Surg 2001;121(9):536—9.

[16] Robertsen K, Kristensen O, Sommer J. Pseudoarthrosis between a patellar tendon ossicle and the tibial tuberosity in Osgood-Schlatter's disease. Scand J Med Sci Sports 1996;6(1):57—9.

[17] Bloom OJ, Mackler L. What is the best treatment for Osgood-Schlatter disease?. 2004 MU Clin Inq 2004; 53(2):153—6.

[18] Rostron PK, Calver RF. Subcutaneous atrophy following methylprednisolone injection in Osgood-Schlatter epiphysitis. JBJS 1979;61(4):627—8.

[19] Topol GA, Podesta LA, Reeves KD, Raya MF, Fullerton BD, Yeh HW. Hyperosmolar dextrose injection for recalcitrant Osgood-Schlatter disease. Pediatrics 2011;128(5): e1121—8. peds-2010.

[20] Krause BL, Williams JPR, Catterall A. Natural history of Osgood-Schlatter disease. J Pediatr Orthop 1990;10(1): 65—8.

[21] Binazzi R, Felli L, Vaccari V, Borelli P. Surgical treatment of unresolved Osgood-Schlatter lesion. Clin Orthop 1993;(289):202—4.

[22] Weiss JM, Jordan SS, Andersen JS, Lee BM, Kocher M. Surgical treatment of unresolved Osgood-Schlatter disease: ossicle resection with tibial tubercleplasty. J Pediatr Orthop 2007;27(7):844—7.

[23] Beyzadeoglu T, Inan M, Bekler H, Altintas F. Arthroscopic excision of an ununited ossicle due to Osgood-Schlatter disease. Arthrosc J Arthrosc Relat Surg 2008;24(9):1081—3.

[24] Eun SS, Lee SA, Kumar R, Sul EJ, Lee SH, Ahn JH, et al. Direct bursoscopic ossicle resection in young and active patients with unresolved Osgood-Schlatter disease. Arthrosc J Arthrosc Relat Surg 2015;31(3):416—21.

[25] Mital MA, Matza RA, Cohen J. The so-called unresolved Osgood-Schlatter lesion: a concept based on fifteen surgically treated lesions. J Bone Joint Surg Am 1980;62(5): 732—9.

[26] Flowers MJ, Bhadreshwar DR. Tibial tuberosity excision for symptomatic Osgood-Schlatter disease. J Pediatr Orthop 1995;15(3):292—7.

[27] Høgh J, Lund B. The sequelae of Osgood-Schlatter's disease in adults. Int Orthop 1988;12(3):213—5.

[28] Jeffreys TE. Genu recurvatum after Osgood-Schlatter's disease: report of a case. J Bone Joint Surg Br 1965;47(2): 298—9.

[29] Lynch MC, Walsh HP. Tibia recurvatum as a complication of Osgood-Schlatter's disease: a report of two cases. J Pediatr Orthop 1991;11(4):543—4.

CHAPTER 13

Sinding–Larsen and Johansson Syndrome

1 BACKGROUND

In 1921, Sinding–Larsen and Johansson described a syndrome in adolescents that associated pain at the distal patella with fragmentation of the patellar pole on X-rays [1]. At one point, Sinding–Larsen–Johansson syndrome (SLJS) was considered as type I bipartite patella [2].

SLJS is a type of osteochondrosis that is histologically similar to Osgood-Schlatter disease (OSD) [3] and caused by repeated traction microtrauma and excessive prolonged stress occurring on a particular skeletal region which is mechanically weak.

This syndrome appears when stress applied during sports activity exceeds intrinsic resistance and repair capacities of the bone tendon junction unit.

SLJS typically occurs in adolescent males between 10 and 14 years of age [4].

The diagnosis is not always obvious. SLJS is used as a general term for all pain conditions at the pole of the patella, but its etiology remains unclear.

In this syndrome, pain is due to abnormal motion of the synchondrosis area that appears mainly after repeated microtrauma in adolescent athletes [4–6]. This theory was based on research in patients with cerebral palsy as a high incidence of SLJS was found in this population ranging from 11% to 28% [7,8], among these spastic patients, 57% had coexisting OSD without a documented injury event.

The histology of SLJS is very similar to OSD, but it is very different from type II or III bipartite patella [3].

Patients can be treated conservatively by immobilization or surgically with loose fragment excision [9]. Pain generally disappears with appropriate conservative treatment, allowing for rapid return to sports activities. Surgical treatment can be considered if the conservative treatment fails [10].

2 CLINICAL STUDY

2.1 Symptoms

The affected child usually complains of pain at the tip of the patella. This symptom could have appeared either progressively or brutally, and in this case, it impairs sports activities.

A history of knee trauma can be found, but most often it is minimal. The onset of pain can follow a live impulse such as a jump or a sprint [1].

This pain is characterized by an increase in intensity during flexion combined with loading of the knee joint.

2.2 Physical Examination

The main clinical features on physical examination are swelling of the infrapatellar soft tissues and knee range of motion (ROM) limitations [3].

Palpation of the patellar tip, forced flexion of the knee, and resisted contraction of the quadriceps awaken the pain.

If the condition is present for a long time, there may be an amyotrophy of the thigh.

In case of acute symptoms, the examiner can note a swelling of the knee with local inflammation signs [5].

Frequently, there is a retraction of the rectus femoris muscle associated with an increased heel-buttock distance (Fig. 13.1).

It is important to examine the tip of the contralateral patella since this affection is quite often bilateral and can remain functionally asymptomatic.

Likewise, the palpation of the tibial tuberosity can reveal pain in relation with an associated OSD since, as mentioned earlier, the association of the two diseases in the same subject is possible [7].

3 DIFFERENTIAL DIAGNOSIS

The differential diagnosis of SLJ disease includes:

3.1 Sleeve Fracture

A history of knee trauma is usually found.

3.2 Osteochondritis Dissecans (OCD)

Pain and swelling of the knee often initiated by sports or physical activity are the most common initial

Knee Pain in Sports Medicine. https://doi.org/10.1016/B978-0-323-88069-5.00008-1

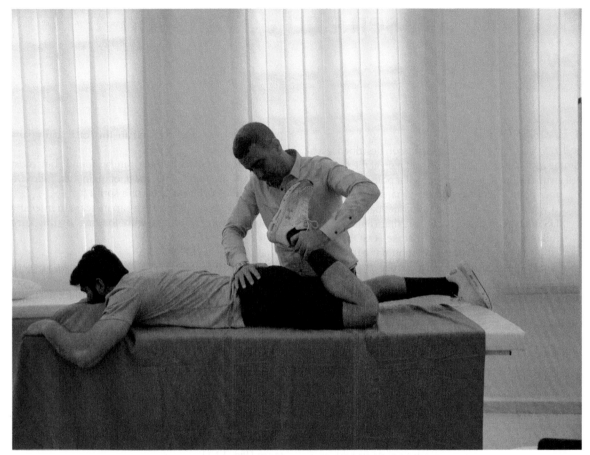

FIG. 13.1 Picture illustration heel-buttock distance assessment.

symptoms of OCD. Advanced cases may present with joint catching or locking.

3.3 Stress Fracture of the Patella

This fracture usually occurs after an increase in the intensity of training. The patient may report a sudden onset of a sharp anterior knee pain.

3.4 Patellar Tendinopathy

Pain in the anterior aspect of the knee is the first symptom of patellar tendinopathy. This pain is worsened by sports activities that require knee extension. On physical examination, there is tenderness on the proximal insertion of the patellar tendon.

4 IMAGING

4.1 Standard X-rays

An X-ray examination may show patellar fragmentation and, in late stages of the disease, calcification of the patellar tendon with possible opacification of the adjacent portions of Hoffa's fat pad [9] (Fig. 13.2).

4.2 Ultrasound

Ultrasound (US) findings are the same as those in OSD. Thickening and heterogeneity of the proximal patellar tendon, especially involving the posterior fibers which attach to the patella rather than pass over its surface to blend with the quadriceps tendon. Focal regions of

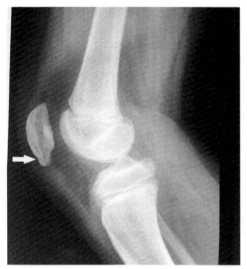

FIG. 13.2 Lateral view standard radiograph of the knee showing patellar fragmentation (*arrow*) in a patient with SLJS syndrome.

hypoechogenicity may be seen in relation to small tears. Cartilage swelling, patellar tendon swelling at its proximal insertion, and patellar fragmentation at its distal pole are possible [6].

4.3 Magnetic Resonance Imaging

Magnetic resonance imaging (MRI) is useful in the assessment of extensor mechanism injuries. In SLJS, the proximal posterior part of the patellar tendon is thickened with high T2 and short tau inversion recovery (STIR) signal. The same type of signal often involves the inferior pole of the patella and in the adjacent fat [11]. This correlates with hypointense signal in these anatomical areas on T1-weighted MRI (Fig. 13.3).

5 TREATMENT

5.1 Conservative Management

5.1.1 Activity modification

Physicians can only act on the triggering factor of cartilaginous suffering that is mainly violent or repetitive contractions of the quadriceps.

In the acute painful phase, therapy is mainly based on rest and abstention from sports activity for at least 1–2 months, particularly football and running that may be replaced by swimming and other sports which exert less pressure on the quadriceps muscle.

5.1.2 Medical treatment

Analgesics and nonsteroidal antiinflammatory drugs (NSAIDs) can be indicated for a short period of time and are useful to reduce painful symptoms.

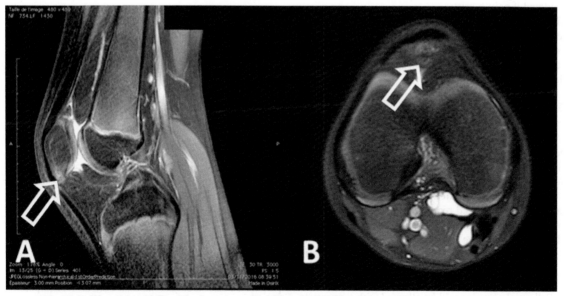

FIG. 13.3 T2-weighted MRI of the knee in sagittal (A) and axial (B) sequences illustrating a fragmentation of the patellar tip and surrounding edema (*arrows*) in a patient with SLJS.

5.1.3 Rehabilitation

A well-established rehabilitation program should address the biomechanical flaws found on examination including functional deficits such as inflexibilities and substitution patterns that compensate for the functional deficits. In SLJS, hamstring and quadriceps tightness and weakness need to be managed [12].

Eccentric strengthening exercises should be given a special importance as the rehabilitation program advances and pain decreases. This type of exercise may provoke pain initially because of the increased stress exerted on the tendon insertion. The final phase of rehabilitation should also incorporate sports-specific tasks and movements.

Knee braces and straps have been used to alleviate pain and to change the force dynamics through the patellar tendon with good results [4].

Modalities such as US and iontophoresis with corticosteroid preparation can also be used to control pain.

5.2 Procedures

Peritendinous injection of corticosteroid has been tried by some authors in cases where noninvasive conservative therapy failed to alleviate pain [3,4]. This procedure can be guided by US to ensure accurate location of the needle. Injection into the Hoffa fat pad has been documented to induce less pain [3]. Hyaluronic acid and platelet-rich plasma (PRP) injections can also be considered if pain persists.

The evolution is usually benign with spontaneous recovery. Thanks to physiological regeneration, full recovery usually takes 12–24 months. When the patella is completely ossified, the pain disappears and complications are rare [13].

5.3 Surgical Treatment

Surgery is indicated in refractory cases or recalcinent PT.

Arthroscopic debridement of the patellar tendon was tried with favorable outcome [14].

During arthroscopy, Hoffa's fat pad behind the patellar tendon is debrided with a shaver. Once the tip of the patella is isolated, it is gradually trimmed away using a motorized reamer until the mobile synchondrosis area is visible. The fragment is released and then excised. The distal end of the patella will be smoothed out to prevent tendon impingement [15].

An intraarticular drain can be left in place for one day. Full weight bearing will be allowed with two canes without an immobilization within the first week. Rehabilitation will be started after one week, with lymphatic draining and exercises to regain joint ROM [16].

6 TAKE HOME MESSAGES

SLJS results from repetitive traction at the inferior pole of the patella in young athletes.

Anterior knee pain is usually of gradual onset and it is worsened by jumping and running activities without trauma history.

On physical examination, tenderness and swelling are frequently found at the level of the patellar tip.

Plain radiographs are usually sufficient to confirm the diagnosis. They may show calcification and ossification in the patellar tendon.

Bipartite patella and a patellar sleeve fracture should be ruled out.

The treatment of SLJS is mainly conservative. Surgical treatment should be reserved for refractory and symptomatic recalcinent cases.

REFERENCES

[1] Sinding-Larsen CM. A hitherto unknown affection of the patella in children. Acta Radiol 1921;1(2):171–3.

[2] Saupe E. Beitrag zur patella. Fortschr Rontgenstr 1921;28:37–41.

[3] Ogden JA, Southwick WO. Osgood-Schlatter's disease and tibial tuberosity development. Clin Orthop 1976;116:180–9.

[4] Bourne MH, Bianco JA. Bipartite patella in the adolescent: results of surgical excision. J Pediatr Orthop 1990;10(1):69–73.

[5] Green JW. Painful bipartite patellae. A report of three cases. Clin Orthop 1975;110:197–200.

[6] Weaver JK. Bipartite patellae as a cause of disability in the athlete. Am J Sports Med 1977;5(4):137–43.

[7] Kaye JJ, Freiberger RH. Fragmentation of the lower pole of the patella in spastic lower extremities. Radiology 1971;101(1):97–100.

[8] Rosenthal RK, Levine DB. Fragmentation of the distal pole of the patella in spastic cerebral palsy. J Bone Joint Surg Am 1977;59(7):934–9.

[9] Iwamoto J, Takeda T, Sato Y, Matsumoto H. Radiographic abnormalities of the inferior pole of the patella in juvenile athletes. Keio J Med 2009;58(1):50–3.

[10] Stocker RL, van Laer L. Injury of a bipartite patella in a young upcoming sportsman. Arch Orthop Trauma Surg 2011;131(1):75–8.

[11] Peace KAL, Lee JC, Healy J. Imaging the infrapatellar tendon in the elite athlete. Clin Radiol 2006;61(7):570–8.

[12] Hawley GW, Griswold AS. Larsen-Johansson's disease of the patella. Surg Gynecol Obstet 1928;47:68–72.

[13] Liddle AD, Rodríguez-Merchán EC. Platelet-rich plasma in the treatment of patellar tendinopathy: a systematic review. Am J Sports Med 2015;43(10):2583–90.

[14] Santander J, Zarba E, Iraporda H, Puleo S. Can arthroscopically assisted treatment of chronic patellar

tendinopathy reduce pain and restore function? Clin Orthop Relat Res 2012;470(4):993–7.

[15] Pascarella A, Alam M, Pascarella F, Latte C, Di Salvatore MG, Maffulli N. Arthroscopic management of chronic patellar tendinopathy. Am J Sports Med 2011; 39(9):1975–83.

[16] Maier D, Bornebusch L, Salzmann GM, Südkamp NP, Ogon P. Mid-and long-term efficacy of the arthroscopic patellar release for treatment of patellar tendinopathy unresponsive to nonoperative management. Arthrosc J Arthrosc Relat Surg 2013;29(8):1338–45.

Instability of the Proximal Tibiofibular Joint

1 BACKGROUND

Instability of the proximal tibiofibular joint (IPTFJ) is a relatively rare cause of knee pain. Patients with this condition typically have no history of trauma or injury. This instability may also be seen in patients with generalized ligamentous laxity. In a few cases, this instability occurs following a recent high energy trauma.

IPTFJ is most commonly seen in patients who practice sports that require violent twisting motions of the flexed knee. It has been reported most frequently in wrestling, parachute jumping, martial arts, gymnastics, skiing, collective ball games, tennis, and skateboarding [1–4].

Recently, it has been reported that IPTFJ may be more common than previously thought and many cases are being misdiagnosed [5].

Instability of this joint may be anterolateral, posteromedial, or inferosuperior.

Mechanisms of the condition include posterior traction on the proximal fibula during knee extension. This traction generates an anterior-posterior motion that is more evident in young children than in adults. A laxity in the joint capsule appears in knee flexion and as a result injuries to this joint generally occur with the knee in a flexed position [6].

Some studies have demonstrated an association between particular anatomic variations of the proximal tibiofibular joint and the potential for developing instability [3,4,7].

Anterolateral dislocation is the most common dislocation of the proximal tibiofibular joint and involves injury to the anterior and posterior capsular ligaments. The dislocation is frequently associated with injury to the lateral collateral ligament [8].

While patients with acute injury usually complain of pain and a prominence in the lateral aspect of the knee, others with microtraumatic dislocation or subluxation report lateral knee pain and instability with popping and blocking which may be confused with lateral meniscal injury.

Symptoms of subluxation are usually treated non-surgically, but for patients with chronic pain or instability, surgical options are considered.

2 CLINICAL STUDY

2.1 Symptoms

It is very important to evaluate the patient's history since this condition may be associated with generalized ligamentous laxity, muscular dystrophy, or Ehlers–Danlos syndrome [4,5,9]. In the latter, most patients are typically preadolescent females and symptoms decrease with skeletal maturity [9].

Subluxation of the proximal tibiofibular joint has also been described in runners who have recently increased their mileage, in patients with history of osteomyelitis, rheumatoid arthritis, and septic arthritis [10].

Typically patients complain of pain and swelling in the lateral aspect of the knee, which is exacerbated by direct pressure over the fibular head [11] (Fig. 14.1).

Some patients may complain of difficulty when climbing stairs [12] and weight-bearing activities may become impossible in many cases because of the pain [9]. Dorsiflexion of the ankle aggravates the lateral knee pain [3]. Knee motion is also very painful and patients may be unable to fully extend the knee [13].

In most cases, no history of trauma is found and the condition is frequently bilateral [8]. Peroneal nerve compression or irritation symptoms may be present especially with posteromedial dislocation [8].

Recurrent or chronic dislocation of the proximal tibiofibular joint can be associated with a wide range of symptoms. Most commonly, knee instability and clicking or popping can be often mistaken for lateral injury of the meniscus [11]. Patients in the chronic stage usually have no difficulty with daily activities, but symptoms may reappear during sports movements that require sudden changes in direction. These movements may produce symptoms of feeling of laxity and the sensation of a prominent dislocation [14].

Knee Pain in Sports Medicine. https://doi.org/10.1016/B978-0-323-88069-5.00003-2

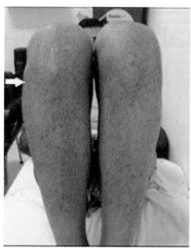

FIG. 14.1 Picture showing swelling in the lateral aspect of the right knee (*arrow*) in a patient with PTFJ instability.

2.2 Physical Examination

Typically a prominent lateral mass is identified in the lateral aspect of the knee, without associated knee effusion [4]. With anterolateral dislocation, there is usually severe pain near the fibular head and along the course of the BF tendon [4].

Tightness of the BF muscle may be present [4].

Pain at the lateral knee aspect is exacerbated by dorsiflexing and everting the foot and with knee extension.

The optimal method for examining the joint requires flexing the knee to 90 degrees, which relaxes the lateral collateral ligament and BF tendon. The knee is palpated for tenderness at this position. Laxity is assessed by translating the fibular head anteriorly and posteriorly while grasping it between the thumb and index finger [12]. This test is positive if the translation reproduces the patient's symptoms (Fig. 14.2).

The Radulescu sign [15] requires the patient to lie prone, with one hand of the examiner stabilizing the thigh and the knee flexed to 90 degrees, the leg is rotated internally with the other hand in an attempt to subluxate the fibula anteriorly.

IPTFJ present in the full extension position of the knee suggests an associated injury to the lateral collateral ligament and posterolateral structures [16].

Examination in all patients with suspected proximal tibiofibular injuries should include an assessment of the integrity of the lateral collateral ligament and posterolateral structures of the knee.

These structures are frequently injured during a proximal tibiofibular dislocation and may cause a problem in the differential diagnosis. In addition, tenderness at the popliteus tendon or BF tendon should be investigated.

3 DIFFERENTIAL DIAGNOSIS

The differential diagnosis for IPFTJ requires excluding a variety of pathologic conditions related to the lateral side of the knee.

3.1 Meniscal Tears or a Discoid Lateral Meniscus

These diagnoses should be suspected in patients presenting with a locking or catching sensation with positive meniscal tests.

3.2 Lateral Knee Osteophytes

Osteophytes are frequently present in case of knee osteoarthritis.

3.3 Intraarticular Loose Bodies

A history of knee trauma is suggestive of the condition, and OCD is also a possible cause of these loose bodies.

3.4 Lateral Collateral Ligament Injury

A history of knee trauma can be found and a feeling of instability can be reported by the patient.

3.5 Biceps Femoris (BF) Tendinopathy

Posterolateral signs are suggestive of this condition and positive tendinous tests help establish the diagnosis.

3.6 Iliotibial Band Syndrome (ITBS)

Lateral knee pain and a snapping a sensation of the knee in runners and cyclists is suggestive of this syndrome. Specific clinical tests confirm the diagnosis when they are present.

4 IMAGING
4.1 Standard X-rays

Bilateral knee X-rays allow a comparison between the two sides and enhance diagnostic sensitivity [17].

The accuracy of diagnosis with the anteroposterior and lateral radiographs alone is reported to be of 72.5% and up to 81.3% when the comparison views are included [18].

Resnick et al. [17] described a line on lateral radiographs that follows the lateral tibial spine distally

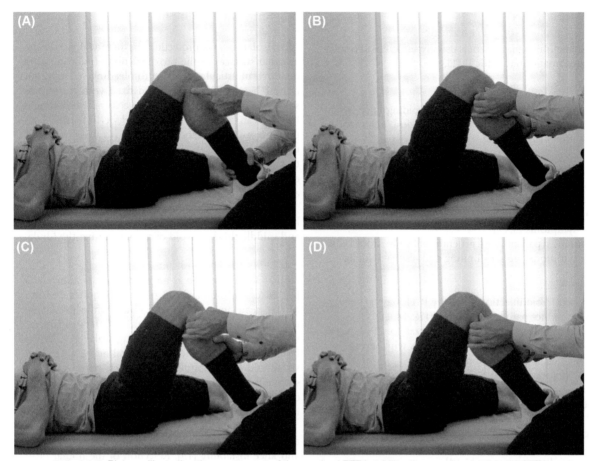

FIG. 14.2 Pictures illustrating the assessment of the proximal PTFJ stability: the examiner locates the PTFJ joint (A), holds the peroneal head between the thumb and the index finger (B), then performs an anterior (C) and a posterior mobilization.

along the posterior aspect of the tibia and defines the most posteromedial portion of the lateral tibial condyle. In a normal knee, this line is found over the midpoint of the fibular head. In anterolateral dislocations, the fibular head will be anterior to this line on the lateral view. In posteromedial dislocations, the whole or most of the fibular head is posterior to this line on the lateral view (Fig. 14.3).

4.2 CT Scan

Axial computed tomography (CT) scan is the most accurate imaging modality to detect injury of the proximal tibiofibular joint with a diagnostic accuracy of 86.3% [18].

This examination is recommended if the diagnosis is suspected on plain radiographs but not clearly established.

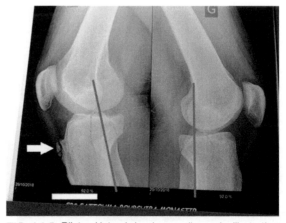

FIG. 14.3 Bilateral lateral view knee radiographs illustrating an anterolateral dislocation of the fibular head in the right knee associated to a fragmentation of the tibial tubercle in relation to OSD sequelae (*arrow*).

5 TREATMENT

5.1 Conservative Treatment

Nonsurgical management is usually sufficient to resolve symptomatic atraumatic IPTFJ.

5.1.1 Activity modification

Activity modification along with avoiding knee hyperflexion is important in the nonsurgical treatment of instability [5].

5.1.2 Rehabilitation

Some authors have found that a rehabilitation program focusing on hamstring and gastrocnemius muscle strengthening may provide some benefit in reducing the symptoms [5,12].

In most patients with generalized ligamentous laxity, the symptoms are self-limiting and resolve with age.

5.2 Procedures

Corticosteroid injections into the PTFJ may be attempted to reduce painful symptoms (Fig. 14.4).

Immobilization in a cylinder cast for 2—3 weeks should be recommended for patients with severe pain to help diminish symptoms [4].

A supportive strap or bandage can be helpful when symptoms of instability persist [13]. The strap is placed 1 cm below the fibular head.

Patients should be advised not to place the strap too tightly because it may precipitate a peroneal nerve palsy. It should be worn as needed during activities that produce symptoms [5,12].

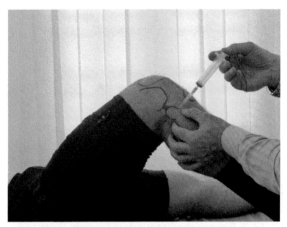

FIG. 14.4 Picture illustrating the needle placement for a corticosteroid injection in case of IPTFJ: the needle is placed between the fibular head and the tibia.

5.3 Surgical Treatment

5.3.1 Arthrodesis

After isolating and protecting the peroneal nerve, the articular surfaces of the proximal tibiofibular joint are denuded of articular cartilage to bleeding subchondral bone. The joint is reduced and fixed with cancellous screws. It is immobilized for 5 weeks and full weight bearing can be started after 8 weeks [12]. Arthrodesis prevents rotation of the fibula, which causes increased rotational stress at the ankle and can frequently lead to pain and instability of the ankle joint [4]. Arthrodesis, therefore, should be avoided especially in athletes and children [14].

If arthrodesis is required, many recommend resecting 1.5 cm of the fibula at the junction of the proximal and middle third to avoid over constraining the fibula.

5.3.2 Fibular head resection

Fibular head resection is an alternative to arthrodesis [4]. Successful fibular head resection requires excision of the head and neck of the fibula while preserving the fibular styloid and the lateral collateral ligament, which is secured to the underlying tibia [13]. When fibrosis is found around the peroneal nerve, a neurolysis should be performed [6]. In fact, peroneal nerve suffering symptoms or palsy in chronic subluxation or dislocation of the proximal tibiofibular joint is one indication for fibular head resection [4].

Unfortunately, fibular head resection has also been associated with the development of chronic ankle pain and knee instability [19]. Resection of the fibular head is contraindicated in both athletes because of the possibility of instability from disruption of the posterolateral corner and in children whose physes are at risk of injury.

5.3.3 Surgical reconstruction

For patients with symptoms of recurrent instability, reconstruction of the supporting structures of the proximal tibiofibular joint can also be done and has shown promising results [14].

Surgical treatment for IPTFJ may include injury to the peroneal nerve [18]. Recurrence of instability and swelling over the proximal fibula have also been described [18].

6 TAKE HOME MESSAGES

IPTFJ is a relatively rare cause of microtraumatic knee pain in athletes.

Patients who practice sports that require violent twisting motions of the flexed knee (wrestling, tennis ...) are particularly prone to IPTFJ.

Patients typically complain of pain and swelling in the lateral aspect of the knee, which is exacerbated by direct pressure over the fibular head.

Antroposterior mobilization and compression of the fibular head reproduce the patient's symptoms.

A special attention should be paid to neurological signs related to common peroneal nerve entrapment.

A comparative plain knee radiographs study aided by the Resnick line has a high diagnostic sensitivity and is usually sufficient to establish the diagnosis of IPTFJ.

Nonsurgical management is commonly sufficient to resolve symptomatic microtraumatic IPTFJ.

Surgical treatment is considered in refractory cases.

REFERENCES

[1] Shapiro GS, Fanton GS, Dillingham MF. Reconstruction for recurrent dislocation of the proximal tibiofibular joint. A new technique. Orthop Rev 1993;22(11):1229−32.

[2] Ogden JA, Southwick WO. Osgood-Schlatter's disease and tibial tuberosity development. Clin Orthop 1976;116:180−9.

[3] Thomason PA, Linson MA. Isolated dislocation of the proximal tibiofibular joint. J Trauma 1986;26(2):192−5.

[4] Ogden JA. Subluxation and dislocation of the proximal tibiofibular joint. JBJS 1974;56(1):145−54.

[5] Semonian RH, Denlinger PM, Duggan RJ. Proximal tibiofibular subluxation relationship to lateral knee pain: a review of proximal tibiofibular joint pathologies. J Orthop Sports Phys Ther 1995;21(5):248−57.

[6] Ogden JA. The anatomy and function of the proximal tibiofibular joint. Clin Orthop Relat Res 1974;101:186−91.

[7] Ogden JA. Dislocation of the proximal fibula. Radiology 1972;105(3):547−9.

[8] Ogden JA. Subluxation of the proximal tibiofibular joint. Clin Orthop Relat Res 1974;101:192−7.

[9] Sharma P, Daffner RH. Case report 389. Skeletal Radiol 1986;15(6):505−6.

[10] Lyle HH. Traumatic luxation of the head of the fibula. Ann Surg 1925;82(4):635.

[11] Veth RPH, Klasen HJ, Kingma LM. Traumatic instability of the proximal tibiofibular joint. Injury September 1, 1981;13(2):159−64.

[12] Sijbrandij S. Instability of the proximal tibio-fibular joint. Acta Orthop Scand 1978;49(6):621−6.

[13] Turco VJ, Spinella AJ. Anterolateral dislocation of the head of the fibula in sports. Am J Sports Med 1985;13(4):209−15.

[14] Giachino AA. Recurrent dislocations of the proximal tibiofibular joint. Report of two cases. JBJS 1986;68(7):1104−6.

[15] Baciu CC, Tudor AL, Olaru I. Recurrent luxation of the superior tibio-fibular joint in the adult. Acta Orthop Scand 1974;45(5):772−7.

[16] James C, Parkes I, Zelko RR. Isolated acute dislocation of the proximal tibiofibular joint: case report. JBJS 1973;55(1):177−80.

[17] Resnick D, Newell JD, Guerra Jr J, Danzig LA, Niwayama G, Goergen TG. Proximal tibiofibular joint: anatomic-pathologic-radiographic correlation. Am J Roentgenol 1978;131(1):133−8.

[18] Keogh P, Masterson E, Murphy B, McCoy CT, Gibney RG, Kelly E. The role of radiography and computed tomography in the diagnosis of acute dislocation of the proximal tibiof ibular joint. Br J Radiol 1993;66(782):108−11.

[19] Draganich LF, Nicholas RW, Shuster JK, Sathy MR, Chang AF, Simon MA. The effects of resection of the proximal part of the fibula on stability of the knee and on gait. J Bone Joint Surg Am 1991;73(4):575−83.

Conclusion

Microtraumatic knee injuries result from mild repetitive biomechanical stress associated with physical activity and exercise that exceeds the tissue tolerance and possibility of regeneration of the affected structure. These repetitive forces applied to muscles, tendons, cartilage, bones, meniscus, and ligaments are all low-energy. Therefore, they can be grouped according to the type of structure that is affected.

Tendinous conditions include PT, quadriceps tendinopathy, ITBS, pes anserinus syndrome, BF tendinopathy, and popliteus tendinopathy. These pathologies occur when the tendons of the respective muscles are exposed to repetitive stress loads. Together, they represent the most frequent etiologies of microtraumatic knee pain. Their incidence among athletes depends on the type of sports. For example, the prevalence of PT in professional jumping-centered sports has been reported to range from 32% to 45% of the concerned athletes. The diagnosis is mainly clinical, based on a well-investigated patient history, positive tendinous tests (for resisted contraction, stretching, and tendon palpation), and specific clinical tests for some of them. When the clinical presentation is not typical, US represents an accessible, low-cost, and noninvasive imaging modality that helps establish the diagnosis. The treatment is mainly conservative and should especially emphasize eccentric strengthening.

Bone, cartilage, and meniscal conditions are all related to intraarticular lesions. They include PFP, OCD, and overuse meniscal pathologies. They are mainly associated with weight-bearing activities and are mainly due to biomechanical imbalances and static abnormalities of the lower limbs. Age is a determining factor in the occurrence of some (overuse meniscal pathologies) and an important prognostic factor in others (OCD). Gender is also an important factor in the development of some of these microtraumatic knee lesions (PFP). The prevalence of these conditions may be very high: almost 25%–30% of all knee injuries seen in sports medicine and up to 40% of clinical visits in the general population for knee problems are attributed to PFP. Clinically, these conditions present as a dull ill-localized knee pain that can hinder the athlete's functional capacities and limit their competition performance. The diagnosis usually requires the use of an adequate imaging modality. MRI is the most accurate examination for the evaluation of these conditions. The treatment of PFP is commonly conservative, while the treatment of OCD and overuse meniscal pathologies frequently requires surgical interventions.

Ligamentous conditions that are responsible for knee pain of nontraumatic origin are quite uncommon in athletes. They include ganglion cysts and mucoid degeneration of the ACL and IPTFJ. Degenerative conditions of the ACL are mainly diagnosed incidentally due to the lack of specific clinical signs and tests that allow their diagnosis. IPTFJ is an important condition to keep in mind when investigating for lateral knee pain etiologies in athletes since it can result in serious neurological suffering of the common peroneal nerve. The incidence of these conditions is relatively low compared to other etiologies involving microtraumatic knee pain. The prevalence of intraarticular ganglia cysts of the ACL is less than 1.33% on knee MRI and less than 2% on knee arthroscopy performed in patients with nontraumatic knee pain. Their diagnosis is commonly aided by imaging modalities, especially MRI which represents the gold standard for evaluating soft tissues of the knee joint including the ligaments. Unlike other knee overuse conditions, the treatment of these entities is mainly surgical, with a good success rate but it does not protect the athlete from reinjury.

Osteochondroses of the knee represent a particular entity that should be primarily considered when investigating microtraumatic knee pain in younger athletes. They include OSD (for the tibial tubercle) and SLJS (for the patellar tip) which share the same pathophysiology, symptoms, and management strategies. Their evolution is mainly determined by skeletal maturity. OSD affects 21% of athletic adolescents and is more frequent than SLJS. The diagnosis of osteochondrosis is mainly clinical. Inspection, palpation, resisted contraction of the quadriceps muscle, and tensioning of the extensor mechanism of the knee are key elements to hold these pathologies responsible for knee pain in this population of young athletes.

Knee bursitis is yet another diagnosis that clinicians should consider. A bursitis is a disorder related to an inflammation of any of the bursa in the knee joint region. It is a common clinical disorder that may lead to functional impairments. For example, anserine bursitis is responsible for 2.5% of medial knee pain in athletes. On inspection, there is often a knee swelling, and a limitation in knee ROM especially in flexion may also be found. US and MRI are imaging modalities of choice to confirm the diagnosis. Topographic forms should be known by clinicians since they may be treated with minimally invasive procedures.

For the majority of these conditions, the treatment approach is mainly conservative. This choice is supported by expert opinions and some guidelines which agree that a well-conducted conservative management strategy is usually sufficient to completely resolve symptoms and avoid their recurrence. Conservative treatment should include some form of activity modification to reduce the stress load on the affected structure and allow for proper healing. Medical treatment especially based on analgesics and antiinflammatories is prescribed in the acute phase of the disease and when an active inflammation is present. Muscle relaxants are helpful in some cases especially when a muscle contracture is present. Rehabilitation is the corner stone for this treatment approach as it helps to address imbalances that have resulted in overuse knee conditions and prevent their recurrence. Stretching, knee ROM, and strengthening exercises seem to be the most appropriate forms of physical therapy. These rehabilitation techniques along with some physical modalities represent a viable option for pain management and performance recovery that allow a prompt return to play.

Minimally invasive procedures are also an option for managing these painful knee conditions. They are mainly represented by corticosteroid, hyaluronic acid, and growth factor injections. Their use should be reserved for a selected group of patients since corticosteroid injections are only useful in patients with certain inflammation and present some risk of tendon rupture, calcifications, and cutaneous atrophy. PRP injections are not a guaranteed success and are still fairly expensive. Besides, there is no scientific evidence to support their use.

Surgical treatment should be reserved to athletes who do not respond well to the conservative approach or present initially with lesions that are known to be irreparable conservatively such as tendon tears. There are no specific guidelines for the choice of surgical techniques and they depend mainly on the surgeon's preferences and the athlete's level.

Return to play is an important issue when dealing with these injuries especially in professional athletes since a premature return to play may aggravate the injury of the affected knee, promote chronicity of the symptoms, or lead to injury of other parts of the body because of abnormal mechanics in running or jumping. This is why the athlete should be involved in the management strategy and encouraged to collaborate with the multidisciplinary team, taking into consideration the athlete's competitive priorities.

Prognostic factors include muscle flexibility and the competition level. Patients with pain at rest or during daily activities may have slower response to treatment than patients with pain only during or after rigorous sports activity. For tendinopathies, patients with identifiable tendinous neovascularization on US tend to have more pain and lower functional scores than patients without neovascularization. Lower functional scores and baseline pain duration and severity in PFP are indicators of poor outcomes in this syndrome.

Knee pain of nontraumatic origin is a frequent complaint in recreational as well as professional athletes. The etiologies for this symptomatology are often misdiagnosed since they require great anatomical and biomechanical knowledge. In fact, it is crucial that the clinician should be able to identify intrinsic risk factors (constitutional abnormalities) and extrinsic risk factors (training errors) which can be modified to prompt recovery and avoid recurrence. Treatment approach has to be individualized and includes actions aimed not only at the athlete but also the training equipment, the training surface, and the resting time. This approach should allow a prompt return to play keeping in mind the competition performance and economic issues for the athletes and their teams and at the same time avoiding premature return to play which can delay healing and promote chronicity and recurrence of the injury. Their outcome depends on the establishment of an early diagnosis and an adequate treatment.

Prevention of nontraumatic knee injuries is also important and requires the intervention of sport medicine practitioners especially the team doctor, the fitness trainer, and the physiotherapist who are close to the athlete and involved in his/her training program and conditions.

Evaluation

CLINICAL CASE NO 1

A 19-year-old female volleyball player presents with mechanical knee pain located to the anterior aspect of the knee that is worsened by prolonged sitting and kneeling. The athlete reports a recent modification in the intensity and frequency of her training as her team is preparing for a national competition.

Q1: What training-related risk factors for knee pain should you look for in this athlete?

A1: Insufficient recovery time between training sessions

Extreme uphill or downhill running, or recent modification of training surface

Use of inappropriate or excessively worn footwear

Q2: Identify the first diagnosis that you suspect in this athlete

A- Posterior horn meniscus tear

B- Instability of the proximal tibio fibular joint

C- Patellofemoral pain

D- Popliteus tendinopathy

E- Iliotibial band syndrome

Answer: C

Q3: List the specific clinical tests that you need to perform to underpin the diagnosis

A3: Vastus medialis coordination test

Patellar apprehension test or Smillie test

Eccentric step test

Waldron's test (Phases I and II)

Clarke's test or patellofemoral grinding test or Zohlen's test

Standard step-down test

Q4: Name the indications of standard x-rays in this disease

A4: Standard x-rays are indicated:

In case of a history of recent trauma, dislocation or surgery, joint effusion.

In patients older than 50 years (to assess for patellofemoral osteoarthritis).

In patients who are skeletally immature (to rule out other causes such as osteochondritis dissecans, physeal injury, or bone tumors).

In suspected cases of bipartite patella, loose bodies, and occult fractures.

Q5: List the corner stones of conservative management in this case

A5: Activity modification

Medical treatment

Rehabilitation

Knee bracing

CLINICAL CASE NO 2

A 25-year-old professional male basketball player complains of a dull knee pain located to the anterior aspect of the right knee that appears in the beginning of a game and disappears after warming up. The pain is worsened when landing from a jump. On clinical examination, patellar tendon tenderness was found in conjunction with a weakness of the quadriceps muscle in the affected side.

Q1: What is the most likely diagnosis in this case?

A1: Patellar tendinopathy is the first diagnosis that should be suspected.

Q2: Provide the adequate clinical test used to assess the quadriceps muscle for weakness.

A2: Functional strength testing of the quadriceps may be performed by asking the patient to perform one-legged step-downs.

Q3: An ultrasound examination was prescribed for this patient. Name the main expected sonographic findings.

A3: Ultrasound may find decreased echogenicity, typically in the deep posterior portion of the patellar tendon adjacent to the lower pole of the patella.

Other common findings on ultrasound include tendon thickening, irregularity of the tendinous envelope, intratendinous calcification, and erosion of the patellar tip.

Q4: Name the most appropriate type of exercise that should be emphasized during the rehabilitation program to strengthen the extensor mechanism of the knee.

A4: Eccentric strengthening exercises should be emphasized to strengthen the quadriceps muscle, the patellar tendon, and the quadriceps tendon.

CLINICAL CASE NO 3

A 30-year-old male amateur weight lifter complains of mild pain located to the anterior aspect of the left knee that appears on weighted leg extension exercises, especially in the deep squat exercise, and resolves after the cessation of this activity. On examination of the knee, there was tenderness localized along the superior pole of the patella and the quadriceps tendon. Quadriceps tendon pain was reproduced by resisted knee extension.

Q1: Identify the diagnosis that should be primarily suspected in this patient.

A1: Quadriceps tendinopathy is the first diagnosis that should be suspected (given the type of the provocative exercise and pain location).

Q2: Name the first-line imaging examination that should be performed to confirm the diagnosis.

A2: Ultrasound is the imaging modality that should be performed.

Q3: Pathognomonic signs of tendinopathy found on this examination are:

A- Muscle atrophy

B- Thickening of the different layers of the tendon

C- Loosening of the fibrillar structure

D- Calcifications

E- Joint effusion

Answers: B, C

Q4: List two types of procedures that can be helpful to manage the symptoms.

A4: PRP injection

Corticosteroid injection

CLINICAL CASE NO 4

A 24-year-old male recreational runner presents with left knee pain of gradual onset that is localized to the lateral aspect of the knee and worsened by downhill running. The pain was initially felt at the beginning of the sport activity and, for 2 weeks, the pain has been present even at rest. Knee varus was found on static examination, and a crepitation was felt while palpating the lateral femoral epicondyle throughout knee flexion and extension.

Q1: Name the most likely diagnosis in this young runner.

A1: Iliotibial band syndrome with bursitis should be suspected (type of sport, pain location, and crepitation).

Q2: List four specific clinical tests that can be used to confirm the diagnosis

A2: Renne's test

The Noble test

The Ober test

The Thomas test

Q3: Name the four rehabilitation techniques and modalities that are useful in the management of this condition.

A3: Manual therapy

The use a foam roller as a myofascial release tool to break up soft-tissue adhesions in the iliotibial band.

Iliotibial band stretching

Quadriceps and hamstring muscles strengthening

Cryotherapy

Q4: A foot insole was prescribed for this patient. Determine the rationale behind the use of his device in this case.

A4: The use of a foot orthosis is justified in this case since an orthosis used to raise the heel in runners may decrease the flexion angle of the knee at foot strike and may decrease symptoms.

CLINICAL CASE NO 5

A 27-year-old woman presents with intermittent pain and swelling in the lower medial aspect of her left knee. She has recently started practicing long distance walking. The symptoms started gradually during the past month and worsened when using the stairs. She reported a history of type 1 diabetes. On physical examination, the patient had a body mass index of 29. On inspection, the affected knee was swollen, and tenderness was present on palpation of the medial aspect. The knee range of motion was not restricted.

Q1: The most likely diagnosis in this case is:

A- Medial knee osteoarthritis

B- Pes anserinus syndrome

C- L3-L4 radiculopathy

D- Medial meniscal cyst

E- Malignant tumor

Answer: B

Q2: Name the most accurate imaging modality that allows to establish the diagnosis.

A2: MRI is the most accurate imaging modality for establishing the diagnosis of pes anserinus syndrome.

Q3: List three physical modalities used in an analgesic purpose for this condition.

A3: Ultrasounds

Transcutaneous electrical nerve stimulation

Cryotherapy

CLINICAL CASE NO 6

A 40-year-old recreational runner presents with dull pain of insidious onset located to the posterolateral aspect of the right knee. The patient gave a history of hamstring injury treated conservatively 2 years ago. The physical examination revealed a painful limitation in the knee ROM, the patient's pain was reproduced by passive knee extension resisted knee flexion and palpation of the distal BF muscle insertion, associated with electrical discharge sensation in the posterior thigh. A recent increase in the mileage was reported.

Q1: The most likely diagnosis in this athlete is:
A- Patellofemoral pain
B- Biceps femoris tendinopathy
C- Pes anserinus tendinopathy
D- Quadriceps tendinopathy
E- Patellar tendinopathy
Answer: B

Q2: An MRI of the knee was performed. Provide three possible abnormalities that can be found in this condition.
A2: Findings include:
Intermediate signal zones on T1-weighted sequences
High signal intensity areas in acute injuries on T2-weighted sequences as a result of surrounding edema.
Intrasubstance fluid signal indicating a partial-thickness tear.

Q3: Determine the anatomic substratum for the reported neuropathic pain (electrical discharge) in the posterior thigh of the patient.
A3: This condition is known as gluteal sciatica and is related to irritation of sciatic nerve branches by tissue scarring related to the biceps femoris tendinopathy.

Q4: Recall the best strengthening way to prevent the recurrence of the lesion.
A4: Eccentric strengthening exercises, such as Nordic hamstring exercises should be recommended in rehabilitation programs to avoid recurrence of the lesion.

CLINICAL CASE NO 7

A 26-year-old female professional tennis player presents with intermittent mechanical pain of the right knee. This pain was mainly located to the posterolateral aspect of the knee. She also reported that running had become painful especially when going downhill. The physical examination revealed tenderness and swelling on palpation of the posterolateral proximal corner of the knee especially the area limited anteriorly by the lateral collateral ligament and posteriorly by the BF muscle tendon. In addition, resisted flexion combined with internal rotation of the knee was painful. When evaluating ROM, the knee could not be fully extended.

Q1: The most likely diagnosis in this case is:
A- Instability of the proximal tibiofibular joint
B- Popliteus tendinopathy
C- External meniscus anterior horn tear
D- Lateral collateral ligament injury
E- Iliotibial band syndrome
Answer: B

Q2: Specific sonographic findings in this condition may include:
A- Hypoechoic collection related to a bursitis
B- Knee effusion
C- Decreased cartilage thickness of the lateral condyle
D- Increased tendon thickness
E- Meniscal irregularities and calcifications
Answer: A, D

Q3: Recall the main three procedures used to manage this condition.
A3: Knee bracing
Taping
Corticosteroid injection

CLINICAL CASE NO 8

A 44-year-old recreational male runner presents with a 2-month history of progressive intermittent mechanical knee pain and stiffness. No sensation of locking or instability was reported. The pain was felt as intraarticular and worsened by extreme knee flexion and extension. On physical examination, the knee was swollen with a slightly limited range of motion. Ligamentous tests for laxity and meniscal tests were negative. Standard x-rays were without abnormalities; especially no signs of osteoarthritis. Magnetic resonance imaging of the knee was performed and showed the presence of an anterior cruciate ligament ganglion cyst.

Q1 Anterior cruciate ligament ganglion cyst appears on MRI as:
A- A fusiform or rounded structure
B- A hyperintense signal on T1-weighted images and hyperintense signal on T2-weighted images.
C- A structure surrounded by a clear boundary
D- Fiber rupture
E- Lobulated structure
Answers: A, C, E

Q2: Underline two differential diagnoses to anterior cruciate ligament ganglion cyst
A2: Knee bursitis
Popliteal cyst

Q3: Name the two imaging modalities that can be used to guide transcutaneous aspiration of this cyst.

A3: Ultrasonography

Computed tomography

CLINICAL CASE NO 9

A 14-year-old soccer player presents with dull intraarticular pain of the right knee that has been present for the past 6 months. The patient did not give a history of trauma but reported several episodes of knee swelling that had responded well to icing and NSAIDs. The pain was exacerbated by exercise and stair climbing. On physical examination, the patient had an antalgic gait, with an external rotation of the knee, an atrophy of the right quadriceps muscle was noted and palpation of the medial femoral condyle at 30 degrees of knee flexion triggered the patient's usual pain.

Q1: The most likely diagnosis is:

A- Patellar tendinopathy

B- Osteochondritis dissecans

C- Osgood-Schlatter disease

D- Sinding-Larsen and Johansson syndrome

E- Popliteus tendinopathy

Answer: B

Q2: Describe the specific clinical test that can be used to help confirm the diagnosis in this case.

A2: The Wilson test consists in bending the knee at 90° then passively moving it to 30° of flexion while rotating the foot medially. If the usual pain occurs during the test and resolves when the foot is rotated laterally, the test is positive. The Wilson test detects only medial condyle lesions and has only positive predictive value. This test is helpful for diagnosis and as a follow-up tool. A sudden increase in pain intensity while performing this test suggests an unstable lesion.

Q3: What is the classification that can be used to assess the type of the lesion and which radiological examination is it based on?

A3: The Bedouelle classification can be used to stage the lesion.

This classification is based on standard x-rays of the knees with anteroposterior and lateral views.

Q4: List three examples of surgical modalities that can be used in the treatment of this condition.

A4: Drilling

Fragment fixation

Mosaic osteochondral transplantation

CLINICAL CASE NO 10

A 32-year-old male basketball player complains of intermittent intraarticular pain of the left knee with a locking sensation, an instability, and a history of multiple effusions. The pain is worsened by knee flexion and landing from a jump. The patient did not give a history of acute trauma. Physical examination findings included medial joint line tenderness, positive McMurray's test, locking, and a palpable clicking when flexing the knee. Quadriceps atrophy in the affected side was noticed.

Q1: The diagnosis that should be suspected is:

A- Instability of the proximal tibiofibular joint

B- Meniscal degenerative tear

C- Sinding-Larsen and Johansson syndrome

D- Osgood-Schlatter disease

E- Iliotibial band syndrome

Answer: B

Q2: Name the main objectives of the rehabilitation program in this patient.

A2: Rehabilitation program should include exercises focused on maintaining range of motion, improving hip and hamstring flexibility, increasing quadriceps and hip strength, and retaining knee proprioception. Recommended exercises include cycling, resisted quadriceps exercises, and squats. Gait correction, whether by exercise or supportive orthoses, may also improve knee function and provide pain relief.

Q3: Name the imaging modality that should be performed to confirm the diagnosis.

A3: Magnetic resonance imaging is the gold standard for meniscal imaging.

Q4: Determine the possible grades of this condition based on this imaging modality.

Magnetic resonance imaging signal changes related to meniscal pathology are graded from grade I to grade III:

Grade I signal change is intrasubstance, globular, and does not meet the articular surface.

Grade II signal change is intra substance, linear, and does not reach the articular surface.

Grade III changes reach the superior or inferior articular surface, or both, and represent a true tear.

CLINICAL CASE NO 11

A 10-year-old gymnast girl presented with a 3-month history of bilateral intermittent pain located to the anterior aspect of the knees. She reported that this pain had occurred during activities especially running and jumping and disappeared with rest. The patient did not give a history of knee trauma. The physical examination revealed bilateral tenderness while palpating the tibial tubercle which was enlarged with thickening of the patellar tendon.

Q1: The most likely diagnosis in this case is:

A- Quadriceps tendinopathy

B- Patellar tendinopathy

C- Sinding-Larsen and Johansson syndrome

D- Osgood-Schlatter disease

E- Patellofemoral pain

Answer: D

Q2: Identify the main expected findings on standard x-rays in this case.

A2: Radiological evaluation may show superficial ossification in the patellar tendon, soft-tissue swelling facing the anterior tibial tuberosity and thickening of the patellar tendon.

An ossification in the patellar tendon may be present.

A fragmentation of apophysis shows that the patient is in the chronic stage.

Q3: Deduce the appropriate attitude in case of intense persistent pain in this patient.

A3: Controlled immobilization should be indicated if the pain is too intense.

Q4: Name the possible surgical treatment modalities for this condition.

A4: Surgical procedures include drilling of the tibial tubercle, removal of the loose fragments, autogenous bone graft and tibial tuberosity excision or sequestrectomy.

MULTIPLE CHOICE QUESTIONS (MCQ)

MCQ 1: Typical symptoms of patellofemoral pain include:

A- Posterior knee pain

B- Locking

C- Catching

D- Clicking

E- Tenderness with fibular head translation

Answers: B, C, D

MCQ 2: In athletes, patellar tendinopathy symptoms:

A- Are usually of insidious onset

B- Are located to the posterolateral aspect of the knee

C- Respond well to conservative management

D- Include quadriceps muscle weakness in the chronic stage

E- Usually require full immobilization of the knee

Answers: A, C, D

MCQ 3: Quadriceps tendinopathy management:

A- Is always surgical

B- Should emphasize eccentric strengthening of the quadriceps muscle

C- May include physical modalities to help alleviate the pain

D- Nonsteroidal antiinflammatory drugs and corticosteroids should always be associated together to optimize their effect

E- Foot orthoses may be indicated in some athletes with static foot abnormalities

Answers: B, C, E

MCQ 4: On physical examination in iliotibial band syndrome cases:

A- Tenderness is usually located to the medial aspect of the knee

B- The examiner should look for varus or valgus of the knee

C- Knee range of motion is usually limited

D- The Noble test is commonly positive

E- Soft-tissue swelling is always present

Answers: B, D

MCQ 5: Pes anserinus syndrome:

A- Is characterized by pain localized to the lateral aspect of the knee

B- Is more frequent in male subjects

C- May be associated with swelling at the medial aspect of the knee

D- Is mainly diagnosed clinically

E- Is always treated surgically

Answers: C, D

MCQ 6: In young athletes biceps femoris muscle tendinopathy:

A- Is frequently associated with other hamstring muscle injuries

B- Mainly consists in tendon tears

C- May be associated with neuropathic pain in the posterior thigh

D- Is a differential diagnosis with avulsion fractures

E- Does not require knee standard x-rays

Answers: A, C, D

MCQ 7: Popliteus tendinopathy:

A- Has downhill running as a risk factor

B- Is characterized by pain localized to the posterolateral aspect of the knee

C- Is often diagnosed in professional runners and triathletes

D- Should be treated with full immobilization

E- Is a differential diagnosis of pes anserinus tendinopathy

Answers: A, B, C

MCQ 8: In athletes with anterior cruciate ligament mucoid degeneration:

A- The diagnosis is mainly clinical

B- Knee pain is typically associated to a restriction of range of motion

C- Locking and grinding sensations may be present.

D- Symptoms do not respond well to nonsteroidal antiinflammatory drugs and physiotherapy.

E- Total resection of the entire lesion is recommended

Answers: B, C

MCQ 9: In case of OCD:

A- Pain is exacerbated by weight-bearing exercise and stair climbing

B- The diagnosis may be confirmed with standard x-rays of the knee

C- Radiographic follow-up is necessary until complete healing is obtained in children.

D- Early physical therapy should be avoided

E- Atrophy of the quadriceps muscle is typically present in the acute stage

Answers: A, B, C

MCQ 10: In older athletes with overuse meniscal pathology:

A- Dynamic ultrasound examination of the knee is the gold standard imaging modality

B- Degenerative tears generally have a complex pattern

C- A positive McMurray test is highly suggestive of a meniscal tear

D- Osteochondritis dissecans is a differential diagnosis

E- A meniscal tear on MRI is a formal indication for surgery even if the patient is asymptomatic

Answers: B, C, D

MCQ 11: Identify the correct affirmations regarding knee bursitis:

A- Para-meniscal bursitis is always associated with meniscal tears

B- Eleven bursae are found within the knee region

C- Pain is commonly worsened by extension

D- Local inflammatory signs are a constant clinical finding

E- Prepatellar bursitis is also known as housemaid's knee

Answers: A, B, E

MCQ 12: Identify the correct affirmations regarding knee bursitis imaging:

A- Standard radiographs have a limited value for assessing knee bursitis.

B- Arthrography is helpful in cases of bursitis that do not communicate with the knee.

C- Ultrasonography can be used to demonstrate the location and extent of bursitis

D- Computed tomography is very helpful in the diagnosis of knee bursitis since it has a high soft-tissue contrast.

E- Magnetic resonance imaging can show the exact location of the lesion and confirm its cystic nature

Answers: A, C, E

MCQ 13: Identify the correct affirmations regarding the treatment of knee bursitis:

A- Local cryotherapy helps to decrease pain and inflammation.

B- Oral steroids are indicated as an initial treatment

C- Physical therapy should include stretching and strengthening exercises

D- Ultrasounds should be avoided

E- Liquid aspiration is systematically performed

Answers: A, C, D

MCQ 14: The differential diagnosis for instability of the proximal tibiofibular joint includes:

A- Lateral meniscus tears

B- Intraarticular loose bodies

C- Lateral collateral ligament injury

D- Patellofemoral pain with patellar instability

E- Posterior cruciate ligament mucoid degeneration

Answers: A, B, C

MCQ 15: In the management of IPTFJ:

A- Immobilization in a cylinder cast for 2−3 weeks is useful in some cases

B- Fibular head resection can lead to knee instability

C- Surgery is essentially needed in patients with generalized ligamentous laxity

D- A tight fibular head strapping on may precipitate a peroneal nerve palsy

E- There is no risk of recurrence after surgical fixation of the fibular head

Answers: A, B, D

MCQ 16: Symptoms of instability of the proximal tibiofibular joint include:

A- Lateral knee pain that is worsened with dorsiflexion of the ankle

B- Peroneal nerve compression or irritation symptoms

C- Neuropathic pain in the plater aspect of the foot (neuropathic pain is located to the dorsal aspect of the foot in case of peroneal nerve compression)

D- The patient's pain is exacerbated with pressure over the fibular head

E- Commonly a knee effusion

Answers: A, B, D

Index

Note: Page numbers followed by "f" indicate figures.

Printed and bound by CPI Group (UK) Ltd, Croydon, CR0 4YY

03/10/2024

01040373-0005